Bergamo Spring Conferences on Haematology

Infections and haemorrhage in acute leukaemia

JOHN LIBBEY EUROTEXT (Paris-Londres)
EDITIONS MÉDECINE-SCIENCES
6, rue Blanche, 92120 Montrouge, France
Tél. (1) 47 35 85 52. Fax. (1) 46 57 10 09

Editeur de la revue «Sang, Thromboses, Vaisseaux»

Rédacteur en chef :
Gérard Tobelem.
Mensuel (10 numéros par an).

Abonnements :
Institutions : 650 F; Particuliers : 380 F; Etudiants : 250 F.

Bergamo Spring Conferences on Haematology

Infections and haemorrhage in acute leukaemia

Proceedings of the Conference held in Bergamo on June 13-14, 1988

Edited by

T. Barbui
A. Falanga
B. Minetti
S. Gorini
G. Tognoni
M.B. Donati

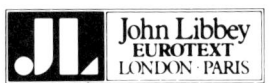

British Library Cataloguing in Publication Data
Infections and haemorrhage in acute leukaemia.
  1. Man. Blood. Leukaemia
  I. Barbui, Tiziano
  616.99'419

ISBN 0-86196-215-X

Editions John Libbey Eurotext
6, rue Blanche, 92120 Montrouge, France. (1) 47 35 85 52
John Libbey & Company Ltd
13 Smiths Yard, Summerley Street, London SW18 4HR, England. (1) 947 27 77

©, 4ᵉ trimestre 1989, Paris.

Foreword

The "Bergamo Spring Conferences on Haematology" are a series of meetings devoted to a multidisciplinary confrontation of new data from fundamental research and clinical practice in haematology.
The first meeting, held in 1987, discussed cellular aspects of haemostasis and thrombosis in the light of information obtained in patients with myeloproliferative disorders; the proceedings have been published in 1988.
The second meeting was held in Bergamo on June 13-14, 1988; it was devoted to physiopathological and clinical problems related to the two major causes of death in acute leukaemia, haemorrhage and infections. The latter complications still represent a challenging problem, despite substantial progress has been achieved in the treatment of acute leukaemias including induction chemotherapy and autologous and allogenic bone marrow transplantation. This book assembles the presentations given at the 1988 meeting.
The next Bergamo Spring Conference will be focused on "Rare Leukaemias" and will be held in 1990. The Proceedings will constitute the third volume of this series.

The Editors

Editors' affiliation

Tiziano Barbui, Anna Falanga, Bruno Minetti. Divisione di Ematologia, Ospedali Riuniti, Largo Barozzi 1, 24100 Bergamo, Italy.
Sergio Gorini. Fondazione Internationale Menarini, Via Settesanti 3, 50131 Firenze, Italy.
Gianni Tognoni. Istituto di Ricerche Farmacologiche «Mario Negri», Via Eritrea 62, 20157 Milano, Italy.
Maria Benedetta Donati. Istituto di Ricerche Farmacologiche «Mario Negri», Consorzio «Mario Negri Sud», Centro di Ricerche Biomediche e Farmacologiche, 66030 S. Maria Imbaro, Chieti, Italy.

Acknowledgements

The support of the "Lega Italiana per la lotta contro i tumori" and of Italfarmaco S.p.A. (Milano, Italy) for the publication of this book is gratefully acknowledged

Contents

Foreword	V
Editors' affiliation	VI

F. Mandelli, R. Latagliata, M.C. Petti
Acute non lymphoid leukemia treatment : an update 1

C.L. Davis, A.Z.S. Rohatiner, T.A. Lister
The importance of infection and haemorrhage in acute myelogenous leukemia 7

E.J. Freireich
Risk factors for hemorrhage and acute leukemia 11

S.G. Gordon, A. Falanga
Procoagulant factors in acute leukemia 19

A. Falanga, M.G. Alessio, R. Consonni, G. Colombi, M.B. Donati, T. Barbui
Disappearance of cancer procoagulant (CP) from bone marrow of ANLL patients after complete remission induction 29

L. Borin, C. Lanzafame, L. Baldicchi, C. Gambacorti Passerini, E. Pogliani, G. Corneo
Cancer procoagulant activity as marker in a case of early cutaneous relapse of promyelocytic leukemia 33

A. Falanga, M.G. Alessio, R. Consonni, G. Colombi, M.B. Donati, T. Barbui
Cancer procoagulant in acute lymphoid (ALL) and non lymphoid leukemia (ANLL) 37

G. Gamba, L. Dezza, L. Ponchio, E. Ascari
Treatment with differentiation agents modifies the expression of procoagulant activities of cultured cells from human leukemias and myelodysplastic syndromes 41

F. Rodeghiero, G. Castaman
Disseminated intravascular coagulation in acute leukemia 45

A. Sagripanti, F. Papineschi, E. Pinori, M. Ferdeghini
Activation of blood coagulation in the blast phase of chronic myelogenous leukemia 65

M. Bazzan, G. Tamponi, A. Fusaro, D. Marranca, C. Tarella
Efficacy of human heat-treated antithrombin-III (At-III) in the management of disseminated intravascular coagulation (D.I.C.) complicating acute leukemia 69

P.G. Canellos
Is heparin necessary in the treatment of acute progranulocytic leukemia ? 73

G. Avvisati, J.W. ten Cate, H.R. Büller, M.T. Petrucci, A. Spadea, F. Mandelli
Tranexamic acid versus placebo in treating the coagulopathy of acute promyelocytic leukemia 77

C. Cordonnier, F. Dreyfus, P. Casassus, V. Leblond, A. Pesce, F. Teilletthibault, P. Colombat, X. Troussard, H. Dombret, M. Gouault, H. Jouault, M. Kuentz, G. Karianakis, J.P. Vernant
Progressive induction for prevention of disseminated intravascular coagulation in acute promyelocytic leukemia : preliminary results 81

P. Rebulla for the Platelet Support Collaborative Group
A clinical trial on the efficacy of leukocyte-depleted blood components in preventing refractoriness to random platelet support : an interim report 89

A. Sagripanti, R. Grazzini, F. Pecori, B. Grassi
Haemocomponents and alloimmunization in the supportive care of leukemic patients 101

C. Giardini, F. Agostinelli, M. Galimberti, P. Polchi, P. Politi, F. Manenti, S.M.T. Durazzi, C. Rossi, D. Baronciani, G. Lucarelli
Blood products for the support of bone marrow transplantation 105

A. Bosi, R. Fanci, A. Orsi, P. Pecile, P. Rossi Ferrini
Isolator lysis-centrifugation blood culture tube analysis in a series of granulocytopenic leukemic patients 109

A. Velardi, S. Cucciaioni, E. Cimignoli, R. Felicini, N. Albi, C. Dembech, A. Terenzi, F. Grignani, M.F. Martelli
Possible mechanisms of late infections in T-depleted bone marrow transplantation : Ig isotype switches leading to selective IgG2-IgG4 subclass deficiency 113

D. van der Waaij, H.G. de Vries-Hospers
Prevention of infections in patients with acute leukemia and granulocytopenia 117

S. Tura, P. Ricci, G. Bandini, E. Calori, L. Albertazzi, G. Rosti, F. Verlicchi, A.M. Foralosso, G. Poletti
Infections in bone marrow transplantation : a comparison between allogeneic and autologous graft 127

D. Caldera, E.P. Alessandrino, P. Bernasconi, M. Boni, E. Orlandi, G. Pagnucco, C. Castagnola, C. Bernasconi
Infectious complications in acute myeloid leukemia in complete remission treated with high dose chemotherapy and autologous bone marrow transplantation 137

G.I.S.I.N. (Gruppo Italiano per lo Studio delle Infezioni nel Neutropenico)
Infection in neutropenic patients. Epidemiology at local institutions : preliminary results of an Italian collaborative study 141

A. Chierichini, S. Nardelli, L. Deriu
Infections in hematologic patients : 10 years of experiences 147

C. Rinaldi, U. Venturelli
Infectious complications in acute leukemic adults : a 4-year retrospective analysis 151

L. Minoli, P. Grossi, A. Malfitano, P. Sacchi, E. Brusamolino, G. Pagnucco
Leukemias and HIV-infection : a case report and a brief review of literature ... 157

G. Landonio, R. Cairoli, I. Shlacht, I. Errante, D. Cipriani
Pneumonia caused by legionnaires' disease in a patient with ALL 163

L. Cavanna, F. Fornari, G. Civardi, M. Di Stasi, L. Buscarini
Sonography and percutaneous aspiration of hepatic abscess in a patient with leukemia 165

E. Orlandi, E. Brusamolino, M. Lazzarino, A. Canevari, E. Morra, G. Castelli, D. Caldera, C. Bernasconi
Febrile and infectious episodes in ANLL patients during induction chemotherapy 169

B. Minetti, B. Marini, F. Gnecchi, C. Farina, M.A. Viviani, T. Barbui
Unusual opportunistic mycoses and concomitant bacteremia in patients with haematological malignancy 173

G. Landonio, A.M. Nosari, L. Gargantini, F. De Cataldo, P. Oreste
Pulmonary and myocardial infarction secondary to arterial occlusion by *Aspergillus fumigatus* in ANLL 177

A.M. Nosari, A. Freyrie, D. Cipriani, M.R. Villa, C. Schiantarelli
Fatal course of cryptosporidiosis in a case of ANLL (FAB : M3) 181

P. Martino, A. Micozzi, G. Gentile, C. Girmenia, R. Raccah, F. Mandelli
The best empiric antibiotic therapy for febrile episodes in patients with acute leukemia 185

G. Capnist, T. Chisesi, A. Vaglia, I. Piacentini, G. Pellizzari, E. Dini
A randomized study comparing imipenem-cilastatin to ceftazidime and amikacin for the treatment of infections in acute leukemia patients. Preliminary results 195

R. Fanci, A. Bosi, G. Longo, A. Bartoloni, D. Aquilini, A. Orsi, P. Rossi Ferrini, F. Paradisi
Preliminary evaluation of ofloxacin (OFL), a new fluorinated quinolone, versus trimethoprim/sulfamethoxazole (TMP/SMZ) in prophylaxis of infections in leukemic patients 201

G. Capnist, T. Chisesi, I. Piacentini, A. Vaglia, G. Pellizzari, E. Dini
Infection prophylaxis in acute leukemia : a comparison of norfloxacin with trimethoprim-sulfamethoxazole. Preliminary results 205

M. Montillo, E. Manso, R. Centurioni, P. Leoni, P.E. Varaldo
Corinebacterium JK infection in an immunocompromised patient treated with teicoplanin 209

P.L. Garavelli
Relationships between serum iron levels and risk of infectious complications in acute leukemia 213

Acute non lymphoid leukemia treatment: an update

F. Mandelli, R. Latagliata, M.C. Petti

Sezione di Ematologia, Dipartimento di Biopatologia Umana, Università «La Sapienza», Roma, Italy

ABSTRACT

In the last 5 years we have unfortunately reached a relative plateau in acute non lymphocytic leukemia (ANLL) treatment. Chemotherapy continues to develop with new combinations which are improving treatment results, even though the proportion of long-term disease-free survivors has only slightly improved. The reason for the non achievement of greater successes are complex; namely:
1. the relatively high number of ANLL patients resistant to standard induction approaches (nearly 10-15% of the cases);
2. deaths due to host (i.e. age) and treatment associated problems;
3. the high risk of leukemic relapse (nearly 60-70%).

The treatment of ANLL falls naturally into two phases: remission induction and post-remission therapy administered in an attempt to eradicate subclinical disease and thus prevent leukemic recurrence. Despite the improvements in remission induction, only a small percentage of patients remains in long-term continuous first remission. Different treatment modalities have been tested. Beneficial effects have been reported by using intensive post-remission chemotherapy. High dose chemo-radiotherapy followed by allogeneic or autologous stem cell reinfusion represent a promising alternative approach especially in patients at high risk of relapse.

KEY-WORDS: ANLL, remission induction, post-remission treatment.

INTRODUCTION

In the past two decades many efforts have been done to improve the prognosis and survival of patients with Acute Nonlymphocytic Leukemia (ANLL). We are now able to achieve Complete Remission (CR) in more than 70% of patients; unfortunately only few patients become long disease-free survivors and most of them relpase with a median CR duration of 10-13 months. Consistent with these results new drugs and new combination are explored to evaluate their efficacy in prolonging CR. Autologous BMT (AUBMT) and above all Allogenic Bone Marrow Transplantation (ABMT) seem to be promising but their exact value in the treatment of ANLL must be evaluated in comparison with intensive chemotherapy.
On the other hand, patients aged over 70 years are commonly excluded from aggressive treatment, since the use of chemotherapy may be seriously limited by a poor

performance status.
Thus advanced age is a major obstacle to very aggressive approaches.

INDUCTION THERAPY

A number of large cooperative groups gave evidence that combination of Cytarabine (Ara-C) and an anthracycline antibiotic is the first line induction therapy, with CR rates ranging from 50% to 80% of ANLL patients (5,7,29,34,40): an overview of these studies indicates the association of 7-day cycles of Ara-C with three days of Daunorubicin (DNR) as the most consolidate schedule.
Addition of a third drug as Vincristine, Cyclophosphamide or 6-Thioguanine to "3+7" schedule is not likely to improve results (10,18). The optimal dose of DNR is also controversial (one to three daily doses of 30-60 mg/m^2), while no difference was observed when DNR was given at the beginning or at the end of the cycle. The optimal mode of administering Ara-C has yet to be established: continuous infusion (200 mg/m^2/day) seems to produce a greater cytocidal effect than i.v. bolus due to the short plasma half-life of the drug (37). Recently a prospective randomized study has shown that 7-day courses of Ara-C were more effective than 5 day courses (31), while no increase of CR rate was achieved with 10 day courses (36).
Rubidazone and Idarubicin seem to be less cardiotoxic and at least as effective as DNR in inducing CR (3): encouraging results by employing induction regimens including 4 days of Rubidazone are reported (22).
Addition of Etoposide to "3+7" schedule might increase the probability of achieving CR in monocytic leukemia (20). Amsacrine, Mitoxantrone and High Doses of Ara-C (HiDAC) have shown an high antileukemic effect, but are currently employed in post-remission treatment or in salvage therapy (2-4-16-26).
Even if monochemotherapy of ANLL belongs to the past, DNR (or Idarubicin) alone for 5-6 days seems to be more effective than "3+7" in promyelocytic leukemia: recently a remission rate of 78% in adult patients was reported from GIMEMA group in a large cooperative study using this drug alone as induction treatment (25).
CR rate is highly age-dependent: using the same intensive induction treatments overall CR rate is less than 50% in patients over 60 years due to the high incidence of induction deaths, while it is over 80% in children (17,21,32,41). Thus should be explored alternative treatments in the elderly: however the impact of those approaches is uncertain.
The use of Low Doses of Ara-C as differentiating agent seemed to be promising, but the overall results are poor and many patients experience marrow hypoplasia (9,30). Because general agreement on the most effective treatment program as to survival and life quality in elder patients is missing, therapy is in many patients individualized according to the clinical characteristics of single patients.
A number of parameters have been suggested to influence CR rate, but only few are well-established prognostic factors (cytogenetic abnormalities, the presence of infections, WBC count over $100.000/m^3$, pre-leukemic syndrome) (12,28,35).

POST-REMISSIN TREATMENT

Once CR is achieved there is no detectable sign of leukemic cells, but minimal residual disease is present and most patients relapse within 1 year: thus, notwithstanding the improvements in remission induction, median CR duration remains disappointingly short and only few patients become long disease-free survivors (11).
Many different treatment approaches have been explored in post-remission phase to improve results. Standard maintenance chemotherapy is based on non-toxic doses of the same or new drugs given over a prolonged period of time (1-3 years) after remission or consolidation therapy: despite the use of maintenance regimens with

great differences in composition and complexity, no major improve in CR duration was observed (29,34,38). Recently the Cancer and Leukemia Group B (CLGB) evidencied that there was no difference in the disease-free survivors rate between 8 months and 3 years of maintenance therapy (31). A randomized study of Italian Cooperative Group GIMEMA after an intensive consolidation phase compared conventional versus intensive maintenance versus no further treatment without difference among these three approaches (29).

Consolidation is based on repeated courses of active drugs, given at doses not producing aplasia, shortly after achieving CR. The Medical Research Council's trial has shown a small advantage (p 0,02) in reducing the number of late relapses, but no significant survival improvement, of 6 courses over 2 courses of consolidation therapy (33). An overview of the present data suggests that consolidation chemotherapy can increase Disease-Free Survival (DSF) percentage, but probably fail to overcome the upper limit of 30% at 5 years.

Two different schedules of intensification therapy, a relatively recent concept in the treatment of ANLL, are been investigated. Early intensification is based on myelosuppressive doses of active agents (1-3 cycles) given immediately after remission; the most important component of this approach are so far HiDAC. Though based on a small number of patients and with relatively short follow-up, some studies (UCLA - St.Louis - CALGB) suggest that early intensification with HiDAC (2-6 g/die for 4-6 days) +/- DNR or Amsacrine may increase the long DSF percentage up to 40% (8,23,42).

Late intensification consists of high-dose chemotherapy with active durgs other than those used in induction in patients who have been in continuous CR for 9-12 months: notwithstanding this approach produced very long CR in some non-randomized studies (6-14), its usefullness seems at present unlikely (27).

ABMT and AuBMT have assumed an important therapeutic role in post-remission treatment of ANLL. ABMT can be performed as an alternative to conventional chemotherapy in first CR to prevent relapse and improve DFS percentage: recurrent leukemia is a common cause of failure in patients transplanted in relapse or in second/subsequent remission. At present data from several transplant centers show a DFS rate of 45-65% of patients in first CR (1,13,19,43). Nevertheless the major limitation of ABMT is that only about 20% of the patients, aged under 45-50 years with an HLA-identical donor, can performe it.

AuBMT should be considered as an alternative treatment and results seem to be very encouraging: Gorin et al reported a DFS of 67% in first remission patients after 4 years, without improvement if marrow purging was performed (15). ABMT role may be different in different subsets of ANLL patients; also in second remission it seems a good consolidation treatment to prolong DFS (24).

At present does not exist any prospective randomized comparison among BMT, ABMT and intensive post-remission chemotherapy in ANLL: recently EORTC, in order to face this problem, has undertaken a randomized study to compare these three different approaches. It is likely that the next years should allow us some conclusions about post-remission therapy of choice.

THERAPY OF REFRACTORY OR RELAPSING DISEASE

Prognosis of patients with refractory or relapsing disease is regarded to be very poor, and alternative therapies including non cross-resistant drugs are recommended: for example HiDAC are able to overcome leukemic cells resistance to conventional doses (2,16,26). CR can be achieved in 20 to 40% of patients with resistant or early relapsed (6 months) leukemia, while CR rate is 50-70% in patients with late relapsed (6 months) leukemia. Unfortunately second remissions are gneerally of short duration: very recently some studies suggested the usefullness of AuBMT as consolidation therapy in these patients after CR achievement (24).

REFERENCES

1. Appelbaum FR, Dahlberg S, Thomas ED, et al (1984). Bone marrow transplantation or chemotherapy after remission induction for adults with acute non lymphoblastic leukemia.
Ann Intern Med 101; 581-8.
2. Arlin ZA, Feldman E, Mittelman A, Baskind P, Sullivan P, Ahmed T (1986). Amsacrine with high-dose cytarabine (HiDAC) is effective therapy for patients with acute myelogenous leukemia (AML) and acute lymphoblastic leukemia (ALL) in relapse (abstract).
14th Internat Cancer Congress, abstr 2847, p 740, Budapest.
3. Berman E, Gee TS, Kempin S, et al (1987). Results of comparative trial of idarubicin and cytarabine in patients with untreated acute non lymphocytic leukemia.
4th International Symposium on Therapy of Acute Leukemias, Rome.
4. Bernasconi C, Lazzarino M, Gherardi S, Amadori S, Mandelli F (1986). Mitoxantrone as single agent in acute refractory leukemia (abstract).
14th Internat Cancer Congress, abstr 1966, p 515, Budapest.
5. Bodey GP, Rodriguez V (1978). Approaches to the treatment of acute leukemias and lymphoma in adults.
Sem Hematol 15, 221-61.
6. Bodey GP, Freireich EJ, Credie KB, Smith TL, Gehan EA, Gutterman JU (1981). Prolonged remission in adults with acute leukemia following late intensification therapy and immunotherapy.
Cancer 47, 1937-45.
7. Cassileth PA, Begg CB, Bennet JM et al (1984). A randomized study of the efficacy of consolidation therapy in adult acute non lymphocytic leukemia.
Blood 63, 843-7.
8. Champlin R (1987). High-dose cytarabine/daunorubicin consolidation chemotherapy for acute myelogenous leukemia.
4th International Symposium on Therapy of Acute Leukemias, Rome.
9. Cheson BD, Jasperse DM, Simon R, Friedman MA (1986). A critical appraisal of low-dose cytosine arabinoside in patients with acute non lymphocytic leukemia and myelodysplastic syndromes.
J Clin Oncol 4, 1857-64.
10. Finnish Leukemia Group (1979). The effect of thioguanine in a combination of daunorubicin, cytarabine and prednisone in the treatment of acute leukemia in adults.
Scand J Hematol 23, 124-8.
11. Foon KA, Gale RP (1984). Acute myelogenous leukemia: current status of therapy in adults; recent results.
Cancer Res 93, 216-39.
12. Fourth International Workshop on Chromosomes in Leukemia (1984). Clinical significance of chromosomal abnormalities in acute nonlymphocytic leukemia.
Cancer Genet Cytogenet 11, 332-50.
13. Gale RP, Kay HM, Rim , et al (1982). Bone marrow transplantation for acute myelogenous leukemia in first remission.
Lancet II, 1006-9.
14. Glucksberg H, Cheever MA, Farewell VT, Fefer A, Thomas ED (1983). Intensification therapy for acute nonlymphoblastic leukemia in adults.
Cancer 52, 198-205.
15. Gorin NC, Harve P, Aegarter P et al (1986). Autologous bone marrow transplantation for acute leukemia in remission.
Br J Hematol 64, 385-91.
16. Herzig RH, Lazarus HM, Wolff SN, Philips GL, Herzig GP (1985). High-dose cytosine arabinoside antibiotics for remission reinduction of acute nonlymphocytic leukemia.
J Clin Oncol 3, 992-7.

17. Kahn SB, Bogg GB, Mazza JJ et al (1984). Full dose versus attenuated dose daunorubicin, cytosine arabinoside and 6-thioguanine in the treatment of acute non lymphocytic leukemia in the elderly.
J Clin Oncol 2, 865-70.
18. Keating MJ, Smith TL, McCredie KB, et al (1981). A four-year experience with anthracycline, cytosine arabinoside, vincristine and prednisone combination chemotherapy in 325 adults with acute leukemia.
Cancer 47, 2779-88.
19. Kersey JH, Ramsay NKC, Kim T, et al (1982). Allogenic bone marrow transplantation in acute non lymphoblastic leukemia. A pilot study. Blood 60, 400-3.
20. Lowenthal PM, Bishop JF, Joshua DE, Mattews JP (1987) Etoposide for remission induction of adult acute non lymphocytic leukemia (ANLL).
4th International Symposium on Therapy of Acute Leukemias, Rome.
21. Mandelli F, Amadori S, Fabiani F et al (1979). Treatment of acute nonlymphocytic leukemia in elderly patients. Results of multicentric study.
Hematologica 64, 331-38.
22. Marty M, Lepage E, Guy H et al (1987). Remission duration in ANLL: a multicentric study of prognostic factors in 461 patients.
4th International Symposium on Therapy of Acute Leukemias, Rome.
23. Mayer RJ, Schiffer CA, Peterson BA et al (1986). Intensive post-remission therapy in adults with acute non lymphocytic leukemia with Ara-C by continuous infusion or bolus administration: preliminary results of a CALGB Phase I study.
Sem Oncol 2 (suppl 3), 84-90.
24. Meloni G, De Fabritiis P, Pulsoni A et al (1988). BAVC conditioning regimen and autologous bone marrow transplantation (AuBMT) in patients with acute myelogenous leukemia (AML) in 2nd complete remission.
Proc Annual Meeting EBMT p 12, Chamonix.
25. Mirto S, Mandelli F, Petti MC et al (1987). Acute promyelocytic leukemia: a perspective GIMEMA study of 84 previously untreated adults.
4th International Symposium on Therapy of Acute Leukemias, Rome.
26. Moore JO, Olsen GA (1984). Mitoxantrone in the treatment of relapsed and refractory acute leukemia.
Sem Oncol 3, 41-46.
27. Morrison FS, Files JC (1985). The effect of late intensification in acute myelogenous leukemia: a Southwest Oncology Group Study (abstract).
Blood 66 (suppl 1), 2052.
28. Passe S, Mike V, Mertelsmann R, Gee TS, Clarkson BD (1982). Acute nonlymphocytic leukemia. Prognostic factors in adults with long-term follow-up.
Cancer 50, 1462-71.
29. Petti MC, Mandelli F, Amadori S, et al (1987). A randomized study of the efficacy of consolidation and post-consolidation therapy in adult acute non lymphocytic leukemia. GIMEMA ANLL 8201.
4th International Symposium on Therapy of Acute Leukemias, Rome.
30. Powell BL, Capizzi RL, Jackson D et al (1987). Low-dose Ara-C for newly diagnosed acute myelogenous leukemia in patients >60 years and for myelodisplastic syndromes.
4th International Symposium on Therapy of Acute Leukemias, Rome.
31. Rai KR, Holland JR, Glidwell OJ et al (1981). Treatment of acute myelocytic leukemia: a study by Cancer and Leukemia Group B.
Blood 58, 1203-12.
32. Reefers J Raynal F, Broustet A (1980). Acute myeloblastic leukemia in elderly patients.
Cancer 45, 2816-20.
33. Rees JKH, Gray RG, Swirts D et al (1986). Principal results of the Medical Research Council's 8th acute myeloid leukemia trial.
Lancet 29, 1236-41.
34. Sauter CHR, Fopp M, Imbach P et al (1984). Acute myelogenous leukemia: maintenance chemotherapy after early consolidation treatment does not prolong

survival.
Lancet 1, 379-82.
35. Schwartz RS, MacIntosh FR, Halpern J et al (1984). Multivariate analysis of factors associated with outcome of treatment for adults with acute myelogenous leukemia.
Cancer 54, 1672-81.
36. Slavin RE, Dias MA, Saral R et al (1978). Cytosine arabinoside induced gastrointestinal toxic alterations in sequential chemotherapeutic protocols. A clinical pathologic study of 33 patients. Cancer 42, 1747-59.
37. Slavin ML, Rohatiner AZS, Dhaliwal HS, Henry GP, Bell R, Lister TA (1982). A comparison of two schedules of cytosine arabinoside used in combination with adriamycin and 6-thioguanine in the treatment of acute myelogenous leukemia.
Med Pediatr Oncol 1 (suppl), 185-92.
38. Toronto Leukemia Study Group (1985). Survival in acute myeloblastic leukemia is not prolonged by remission maintenance or early reinduction chemotherapy (abstract).
Blood 66 (suppl 1), 210.
39. Toronto Leukemia Study Group (1986). Results of chemotherapy for unselected patients with acute myeloblastic leukemia: effect of exclusion on interpretation of results.
Lancet 1, 786-8.
40. Yates J, Glidewell O, Wiernik P et al (1982). Cytosine arabinoside with daunorubicin or adriamycin for therapy of acute myelocytic leukemia: a CALGB study.
Blood 60, 865-8.
41. Weinstein JH, Maye JR, Rosenthal DS et al (1983). Chemotherapy for acute myelogenous leukemia in children and adults: VAPA up date.
Blood 62, 315-9.
42. Wolff SN, Marion J, Stein RS et al (1985). High-dose cytosine arabinoside and daunorubicin as consolidation therapy for acute non lymphocytic leukemia in first remission: a pilot study. Blood 65, 1407-11.
43. Zwaan FE, Hermans J, Barrett AJ et al (1984). Bone marrow transplantation for acute non lymphoblastic leukemia: a survey of the European group for Bone Marrow Transplantation.
Br J Hematol 56, 645-53.

The importance of infection and haemorrhage in acute myelogenous leukaemia

C.L. Davis, A.Z.S. Rohatiner, T.A. Lister

Medical Oncology, St. Bartholomew's Hospital, London, U.K.

Infection and haemorrhage are inevitable features of the natural history of acute myelogenous leukaemia (A.M.L.) and are by far the commonest causes of death in untrated patients (Scott RB, 1957; Tivey H, 1955).
Intensive combination chemotherapy, supported by antibiotic and blood products, results in complete remission being attained in up to three-quarters of those treated. A significant proportion of these patients are curable (Beguin Y et al., 1985; Rees JKH et al., 1986; Champlin R et al., 1987). The objective of chemotherapy in acute leukaemia is to achieve temporary aplasia and therefore, the risk of fatal infection and haemorrhage is particularly high during treatment. Measures can be taken both to prevent this sequelae and to treat them promptly but despite this, infection and haemorrhage prevent complete remission being achieved in a considerable number of patients (Estey EH et al., 1982).

The results of the treatment of newly diagnosed, patients with AML at St. Bartholomew's Hospital, London can be used to support this premise (Rohatiner AZS et al., 1988; Tucker J et al., 1988). Between 1978 and 1986, 275 patients aged between 15 and 76 years received combination chemotherapy with curative intent. Almost all younger patients but only 76% of older patients were intensively treated (88/115). 68% of the group (187/275) were under the age of 60 at diagnosis and 32% (88/275) were older. The precise details of the chemotherapy regimes employed will not be discussed here.

All patients were nursed on open wards, prophylactic non-adsorbable antibiotics (Framycetin, Nystatin and Colistin) were prescribed for the duration of therapy (Storring RA et al., 1977), although not always taken, and combinations of intravenous broad-spectrum antibiotics were administered, after appropriate investigation, if there was any indication of infection. These antibiotics were changed on the basis of microbiological sensitivities and the clinical status of the patient. Single donor platelet concentrates were given both prophylactically, to maintain the platelet count greter than $20 \times 10^9/l$, and whenever bleeding occurred. Patients with promyelocitic leukaemia received platelet transfusions to maintain the platelet count greter than $50 \times 10^9/l$ during remission induction.

The overall complete remission rate was 55% (143/275) -complete remission was not achieved in 132 cases, 69/187 (37%) younger and 63/88 (72%) older patients, and this was due to either supportive care failure or resistant disease. These rates are similar to those from other centres (Brincker H, 1985; Curtis JE et al., 1979). Supportive care failure was defined as death from infection or haemorrhage occurring within six weeks of presentation after one of two cycles of treatment. This was the predominant cause of failure to achieve complete remission and accounted for 45/69 (65%) of the younger and 38/63 (60%) of the older non-remitters. Patients in whom the cellularity and blast cell count in the bone marrow had not been substantially reduced after two cycles of therapy were considered to have resistant disease and this accounted for failure to achieve complete remission in 19/66 younger (27.5%) and 21/63 (33.3%) older patients.

Overall, 75/83 (90%) of these patients dying of supportive care failure died of infection and only 8/83 of haemorrhage, an intracerebral bleed in most cases. Further analysis reveals that 40/45 of younger and 35/38 older patients died of infection, the median time from the start of chemotherapy to death being 17 days. 4/45 younger and 3/38 older patients died of bleeding, the median time to death being 6 days -3 of this 8 patients had promyelocytic leukaemia.

Thus, the lower remission rate in older patients, 28% as opposed to 63%, is mainly due to the greater number of deaths during the hypoplastic period, before complet remission could be achieved. Provided that remission could be achieved in the older patients, the frequency of relapse was no greater than that in younger patients and so the worse survival figures for the older patients are directly attributable to a greater numbers of deaths from infection.

Infection is the major obstacle in the prevention of achievement of complete remission in adult patients with AML whilst haemorrhage is almost irrelevant. It is to be hoped that the use of newer antibiotic regimes may decrease this figure still further so that ultimately, the only important factor preventing the attainment of complete remission in AML will be resistant disease.

CAUSES OF FAILURE TO ACHIEVE COMPLETE REMISSION IN INTENSIVELY TREATED PATIENTS

	Younger patients	Older patients
Resistant disease	19	21
Death due to infection	40	35
Death due to haemorrhage	5	3
Death due to other causes	5	4
	69	63

REFERENCES

Beguin Y, Bury J, Fillet G, Lennes G. Treatment of acute non-lymphocytic leukaemia in young and elderly patients. Cancer 1985; 56:2587.

Brincker H. Estimate of overall treatment results in acute leukemia on age-specific rates of incidence and of complete remission. Cancer Treat Rep 1985; 69: 5.

Champlin R, Gale RP. Acute myelogenous leukemia: recent advances in therapy. Blood 1987; 69:1551.

Curtis JE, Till JE, Messner HA et al. Comparison of outcomes and prognostic factors for two groups of patients with acute myeloblastic leukemia. Leukemia Res 1979; 3: 409.

Estey EH, Keating MJ, McCredie KB, Bodey GB, Freireich EJ. Causes of initial remission induction failure in acute myelogenous leukemia. Blood 1982; 60:309.

Rees JKH, Gray RG, Swirsky D et al. Principal results of the Medical Research Council's 8th Acute Myeloid Leukaemia trial. Lancet 1986; 2:1123-1241.

Rohatiner AZS, Gregory WM et al. Short Term Therapy for AML. J Clin Onc 1988; 6, No2: 218-226.

Scott RB. Leukaemia. Lancet 1957; i:1053.

Storring RA, Mc Elwain TJ, Jameson B et al. Oral non-absorbed antibiotics prevent infection in acute non-lymphoblastic leukaemia. Lancet 1977; 2: 837-840.

Tivey H. The natural history of untreated acute leukaemia. Ann NY Acad Sci 1955; 60:32.

Tuckr J, Amess JAL, Gregory WM et al. Acute myeloid leukaemia in elderly adults. Haemat Oncol 1988; in press.

Risk factors for hemorrhage and acute leukemia

E.J. Freireich

University of Texas, M.D. Anderson Cancer Center, 1515 Holcombe Blvd., Houston, Texas 77030, U.S.A.

ABSTRACT

Hemorrhage remains a major cause of morbidity and mortality in leukemia. Improved methods for collection, storage and determining compatibility between donor and recipient for platelet replacement is a major component of improving the management of these complications. However the importance of consumptive coagulopathy is increasingly appreciated. Infection is a major contributor to this syndrome. Hyperleukocytosis, particularly in acute leukemia, is another important variable. Aggressive treatment of hypofibrinogenemia and thrombocytopenia are an essential part of the management of leukemia and further improvements in the management of these hemorrhagic complications should improve the overall prognosis.

Keyword: Hemorrhage, platelets, transfusion, disseminated intravascular coagulation (D.I.C.), hypofibrinogenemia

Prior to 1960, hemorrhage was the leading cause of fatality in patients with acute leukemia. More than two-thirds of patients had hemorrhage as a significant contribution to mortality and over 20% had hemorrhage as the principle cause of death (Hersh, 1965). The role of thrombocytopenia in this hemorrhagic diathesis was appreciated when quantitative phase microscopic counting of platelets became technically possible (Gaydos, 1962). It was demonstrated that the risk of hemorrhage is directly related to the degree of thrombocytopenia. Petechial hemorrhage and gross bleeding was rarely observed when platelet counts exceeded 20,000 per ul and this observation stimulated renewed investigation of allogeneic platelet replacement. The observation that replacement of blood loss with fresh whole blood was associated with a significant reduction in hemorrhage focused attention on the need for more effective methods for the collection of platelets (Freireich, 1959).

PLATELET REPLACEMENT TRANSFUSION

The adaptation of the closed plastic blood collecting systems to allow the collection of two units, that is, the platelets from two full units of blood followed by centrifugal separation of platelets and return of the red cells to the donors opened a whole new field of replacement therapy (Kliman, 1961). The platelets from up to four units of whole blood which represent approximately 3 to 4×10^{11} platelets can be collected from a single donor in a single procedure with current technology utilizing continuous flow blood cell separating equipment or intermittent flow collecting systems (Hester, 1987).

It was subsequently demonstrated that such platelet rich plasma could effectively elevate the circulating platelet concentration by 12,000 per ul per 10^{11} platelets injected per sq. m body surface area (Freireich, 1963). When such replacement platelet transfusion was incorporated into overall patient care, a major decrease in the frequency of hemorrhage was documented.

Despite aggressive replacement of platelets from allogenic donors, hemorrhage remains an important contributor to morbidity and mortality in acute leukemia (Chang, 1976).

FACTORS RELATED TO THE EFFECTIVENESS OF PLATELET TRANSFUSION

An important factor in determining the effectiveness of platelet transfusion is the quality of the platelets transfused. Platelet preparations may vary greatly in quality, unless careful attention is given to the preparation of concentrates to avoid major platelet clumping and to assure that the platelets are fresh, that is, as close to donation as possible. Platelets which are maintained in an adequate amount of plasma at room temperature and continuously agitated have the best *in vitro* performance, however, storage for periods of 24 to 48 hours results in significant decrease in the viability of the platelet preparations (Vallejos, 1973).

Another important variable relates to isosensitization to platelet specific antigens. A major component of this can be corrected by use of the HLA tissue typing antigens. The practice of selection of relatives for platelet donations improves the quality and avoids sensitization. In isosensitized donors, HLA tissue typing of donors and recipients has proven useful for donor selection. There are a number of cross matching procedures that have been developed, although general application remains to be of proven usefulness. Finally, choosing donors for single donor donations on a sequential basis often allows the identification of compatible donors. An exciting new development in avoiding isosensitization is the use of autologous platelets in circumstances where severe thrombopenia can be anticipated. The current methods for in vitro preservation by freezing of platelets are sufficiently well developed that the patient's own platelets can be stored for use during periods of thrombocytopenia (Schiffer, 1987).

Splenomegaly is an important clinical variable that is occasionally overlooked and it is documented that in the presence or absence of specific isosensitization, the presence of the spleen contributes to a poor response to replacement transfusion (Flatow, 1966; Bishop, 1988).

THE EFFECT OF LEUKEMIA ON THE HEMORRHAGIC DIATHESIS

When a patient with leukemia, particularly acute leukemia, develops a "blast crisis" characterized by a rapidly rising and greatly elevated number of circulating leukemic cells, a unique hemorrhagic diathesis results. Intracerebral leukostasis followed by proliferation of leukemic cells in vessels with destruction of arteries results in arteriole hemorrhage in major organs. It was first reported to be associated with intracerebral hemorrhage (Freireich, 1960). It is now appreciated that pulmonary leukostasis with a picture resembling pneumonia is frequently caused by hemorrhage associated with hyperleukocytosis. These patients have a significantly lower probability of achieving a complete remission and have an significantly increased frequency of the signs of disseminated intravascular coagulation, that is, an accompanying hypofibrinogenemia and elevated fibrin split products "Table 1".

TABLE 1

85 AML Patients; WBC > 100,000 per µl

% (p)

	CR	Fail	Total
Patients	56	44	100
Pulmonary Leukostasis	23	62 (.01)	40
D.I.C. Pre Rx	10	24 (>.05)	16

The major cause for this poor response is death during early treatment. Hemorrhage into the lungs and central nervous system is the major cause of this early mortality "Table 2" (Ventura, 1988).

TABLE 2

Cause of Death

37 Patients, WBC > 100,000

	%
Death During 1st Course	46
Pulmonary Hemorrhage	88
CNS Hemorrhage	29

In patients with acute promyelocytic leukemia, there is a substantially higher frequency of disseminated intravascular coagulation at presentation "Table 3" (Gould, 1988). Patients with promyelocytic (M_3) leukemia have a lower frequency of response as a result of this complication.

TABLE 3

Patients with Acute Myeloblastic Leukemia, # (%)

Fibrinogen mgm %	M_3	Other	Total
< 200	25 (66)	66 (14)	91 (17)
> 200	13 (34)	405 (86)	418 (82)
Total	38	471	509 (100)

Recently, it has been observed that D.I.C. at presentation also occurs in other forms of acute myeloblastic leukemia and as with promyelocytic leukemia, the presence of a fibrinogen level below 200 mg percent is associated with a lower frequency of achieving complete remission and an increased earlier mortality. An important new finding, is that, hypofibrinogenemia itself has proven to be prognostically important. The appreciation of the importance of D.I.C. and hypofibrinogenemia has led to early efforts to aggressively correct this deficiency. We have studied a small number of patients employing plasma exchange transfusion at the outset, in an effort to correct this complication. Preliminary results suggest that this is a promising approach to this complication.

RESUME

Prior to 1960, hemorrhage was the leading cause of fatality in patients with acute leukemia. More than two-thirds of patients had hemorrhage as a significant contribution to mortality and over 20% had hemorrhage as the principle cause of death. While many factors contribute to this complication, the dominant role of thrombocytopenia was recognized and the introduction of allogeneic platelet replacement transfusion sharply reduced the risk of hemorrhage. Despite rapid advances in techniques for collection, storage, typing and transfusion of platelets, hemorrhage remains a major contributory factor to mortality and morbidity. Ten to 15% of patients have hemorrhage as their principle cause of death and another 15% have major morbidity resulting from hemorrhage. An important cause of this persistent problem with bleeding is resistance to platelet transfusion from allogeneic donors. A major component in this is isosensitization resulting from prior exposure to blood products. Yet, appropriate cross matching techniques do not exist and replacement from single donors and from HLA related siblings provides only a partial solution to the problem of isosensitization.

Another factor in resistance to platelet replacement is consumptive coagulopathy. This is particularly striking in acute promyelocytic leukemia. In this disease, disseminated intravascular coagulation (DIC) presents with low plasma fibrinogen, high fibrin split products. The hemorrhagic diathesis results in 25% to 30% mortality during the early phases of treatment.

Aggressive replacement of procoagulants and platelets are effective in some but not regularly effective. Preliminary data involving exchange transfusion of patients with DIC suggest this is a promising approach to the problem.

In other patients with acute granulocytic leukemia, the level of plasma fibrinogen is an important predictor for response to treatment and for hemorrhagic complications. Patients with plasma levels below 200 mgm %, have an increased risk of hemorrhagic complications. If aggressive replacement of procoagulants and platelets demonstrates rapid consumption of procoagulants associated with elevated split products then plasma exchange is another approach to this important complication. Hyperleukocytosis, particularly, circulating leukocyte counts in excess of 100,000 per ul, is frequently associated with intravascular leukostasis and contributory to hemorrhagic complications. While intracerebral hemorrhage was the first of these complication to be recognized, pulmonary leukostasis has emerged as a major cause of respiratory insufficiency often misdiagnosed as pneumonia. Rapid lowering by pheresis of the circulating leukocyte count can result in reversal of these complications and prevention of the attendant hemorrhagic complications.

Hemorrhage remains a major contributor to morbidity and mortality in acute leukemia. In addition to accelerated consumption initiated by the leukemic process, the complication of infection greatly aggravates these problems. Innovative approaches to consumptive coagulopathy are proposed in hopes of controlling these major complications.

REFERENCES

Bishop, J.F., McGrath, K., Wolf, M.M., Matthews, J.P., De Luise, T., Holdsworth R., Yuen, K., Veale, M., Whiteside, M.G., Cooper, I.A., Szer, J.(1988): Clinical factors influencing the efficacy of pooled platelet transfusions. Blood 71(2), 383-387.

Chang, H.Y., Rodriguez, V., Narboni, G., Bodey, G.P., Luna, M.A., and Freireich, E.J (1976): Causes of death in adults with acute leukemia. Medicine 55, 259-268.

Flatow, F.A., and Freireich, E.J (1966): The effect of splenectomy on response to platelet transfusion in three patients with aplastic anemia. N. Engl. J. Med. 274, 242-248.

Freireich, E.J, Kliman, A., Gaydos, L.A., Mantel, N., and Frei, E. III (1963): Response to repeated platelet transfusions from the same donor. Ann. Intern. Med. 59, 277-287.

Freireich, E.J, Schmidt, P.J., Schneiderman, M.A., and Frei, E. III (1959): A comparative study of the effect of transfusion of fresh and preserved whole blood on bleeding in patients with acute leukemia. N. Engl. J. Med. 260, 6-11.

Freireich, E.J., Thomas, L.B., Frei, E. III, Fritz, R.D., Forkner, C.E., Jr. (1960): A distinctive type of intracerebral hemorrhage associated with "blastic crisis" in patients with leukemia. Cancer 13, 146-154.

Gaydos, L.A., Freireich, E.J, and Mantel, N. (1962): The quantitative relation between platelet count and hemorrhage in patients with acute leukemia. N. Engl. J. Med. 266, 905-909.

Gould, J., Keating, M., Kantarjian, H., Estey, E., Hester, J., McCredie, K., Freireich, E.J (1988): The prognostic significance of pretreatment fibrinogen levels in acute myelogenous leukemia. (Submitted for publication).

Hersh, E.M., Bodey, G.P., Nies, B.A., and Freireich, E.J (1965): Causes of death in acute leukemia. A ten year study of 414 patients. J. Amer. Med. Assoc. 193, 105-109.

Hester, J.P., Ventura, G.J., and Boucher, T.(1987): Platelet concentrate collection in a dual-stage channel using computer--generated algorithms for collection and prediction of yield. Plasma Ther. Transfus. Technol. 8, 377-385.

Kliman, A., Gaydos, L.A., Schroeder, L.R., and Freireich, E.J (1961): Repeated plasmapheresis of blood donors as a source of platelets. Blood 18, 303-309.

Schiffer, C.A. (1987): Management of patients refractory to platelet transfusion — An evaluation of methods of donors selection. Prog. in Hematol. 15, 91-113.

Vallejos, C.S., Freireich, E.J, Brittin, G.M., and De Jongh, D.S. (1973): Effects of platelets stored at 22° C for 24 hours in patients with acute leukemia. Blood 42, 565-570.

Ventura, G.J., Hester J.P., Smith, T.L., and Keating, M.J.(1988): Acute myeloblastic leukemia with hyperleukocytosis: Risk factors for early mortality in induction. Amer. J. Hematol. 27, 34-37.

Procoagulant factors in acute leukemia

S.G. Gordon, A. Falanga

*University of Colorado Health Sciences Center, Denver, CO 80262, USA
and Divisione di Ematologia, Ospedali Riuniti di Bergamo, Bergamo, Italy*

ABSTRACT

Patients with acute non-lymphocytic leukemia, particularly those with promyelocytic leukemia, frequently have either bleeding or clotting problems. This discussion focuses on the initiation of coagulation by tissue factor and cancer procoagulant. A chronic low grade activation of the coagulation system may cause a depletion of clotting factors or inhibitors that can lead to a bleeding diathesis; if higher level of activation occurs, it can lead to a clotting diathesis. Tissue factor is a membrane glycoprotein that is a factor VII receptor. It is associated with all normal and malignant cells. Its amino acid sequence reveals a 219 external segment with 3 glycosylation sites, 4 half-cystines and 3 tryptophan-lysine-serine tripeptides that may bind factors VII, IX and X. There is a 23 amino acid transmembrane segment and a 22 amino acid intracellular segment that may participate in metabolic control of tissue factor activity. Cancer procoagulant was originally described associated with solid tumor cells but recent studies have demonstrated that it is also associated with ANLL cells. Bone marrow or peripheral blood cells were extracted and assayed for procoagulant activity. Their factor VII independent activity ranged from 0 to 100% in M1, M2, M3 cytologic subtypes; M4 had less and M5 had no factor VII independent activity. The M2 and M3 extracts directly activated factor X in a 2 stage clotting assay. The M1, M2 and M3 extracts were inhibited by iodoacetamide and $HgCl_2$ (cysteine proteinase inhibitors) while the M5 and, to a lesser extent, the M4 extracts were inhibited by concanavalin A, a tissue factor inhibitor. Thus, ANLL cells have both tissue factor and cancer procoagulant for the initiation of coagulation.

KEY WORDS

Acute Non-Lymphocytic Leukemia, Procoagulants, Tissue Factor, Cancer Procoagulant, Prothrombinase Complex, Blood Coagulation

INTRODUCTION

Coagulation abnormalities associated with acute leukemia present in several forms with a spectrum of clinical severities. Usually patients have a bleeding or hemorrhage problems. Some patients have overt coagulopathies with disseminated intravascular coagulation and deep vein thrombosis. Most patients are thrombocytopenic and slightly anemic. Most of these clinical pictures are associated, directly or indirectly with the activation of the coagulation cascade by procoagulant factors from leukemia cells.

Thrombocytopenia and anemia are caused by an overproduction of the malignant leukemia cells that displaces the production of normal platelets and red cells by the bone marrow, resulting in a depressed production capacity for the normal cellular components of the blood (Linman, 1978). In addition, circulating platelets become activated by the coagulation proteinases (thrombin), resulting in the enhanced removal of platelets from the blood (Bratt, 1985a). Decreasing platelet activation and removal by decreasing the activity of the coagulation cascade would provide partial relief of the thrombocytopenia associated with acute leukemia.

The activation of the coagulation cascade is responsible for both the bleeding/hemorrhage and coagulopathy seen in acute leukemia. Low grade activation of the coagulation system results in consumption of both coagulation and anti-coagulation factors (Bratt, 1985b). This activation is frequently sub-clinical and presents with few, if any, clinical symptoms of a coagulopathy but the end result is a bleeding diathesis. Due to differences in rates of consumption and synthesis of these factors, there is no general agreement about the coagulation factor profile at the onset of bleeding problems. Deficient factors include fibrinogen, factor XIII and protein C (Berild, 1987; Egbring, 1977). Consumption (destruction) of coagulation factors like fibrinogen is also attributed to the release of proteinases from cells that are destroyed by either the disease process or therapeutic treatments of the disease. For example, chemotherapy of acute leukemia causes the cytolysis of leukemic cells and normal monocytes, resulting in the release of cathepsins and elastase into the circulation. Elastase partially degrades fibrinogen to an unclottable protein and facilitates a functional deficiency of fibrinogen (Marlar, 1985; Bauer, 1984; Sterrenberg, 1985). Other proteinases may cause a similar problem.

The expression of procoagulant activity increases, it facilitates higher levels of activity within the coagulation cascade and the clinical presentation shifts from bleeding and hemorrhage to clotting and thrombosis. Acute promyelocytic leukemia (APL) is the most common form of ANLL that presents with overt coagulopathy; others forms present with clotting problems at a less frequently.

Procoagulant factors, particularly those associated with APL, have been the focus of much research for more that two decades. However, new discoveries within the last few years have provided important information that may help explain the clinical observation in acute leukemia. The procoagulants that appear to play a role in the coagulation abnormalities of acute leukemia include tissue factor and cancer procoagulant. In addition, factor Va receptor may represent a significant participant in the activity of the coagulation system in these clinical problems. All these factors have been identified as participants in the coagulation abnormalities associated with solid malignancies.

Figure 1 shows a schematic diagram of a major part of the classic coagulation cascade with a few additions. One addition is the activation of factor IX by tissue factor and factor VIIa. The second addition is the activation of factor X by cancer procoagulant. Over the past few years, it has become apparent that there are several unique aspects to the enzymology of the coagulation system; primarily the fact that many of the reactions take place on cell surfaces. There are three "cell surface" reactions, tissue factor-factor VII activation of either factor IX or factor X, factor VIIIa-factor IXa activation of factor X and factor V-factor Xa activation of prothrombin. The two that are important for this discussion are the tissue factor and factor V reactions.

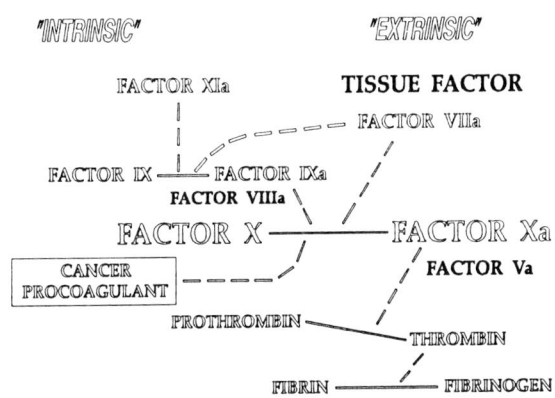

Figure 1
A Schematic Diagram of the Coagulation System. Two notable differences from the classic scheme are the activation of factor IX by tissue factor-factor VIIa and the addition of cancer procoagulant. The membrane co-factors for the assembly of the activation complexes are represented in solid letters. The intrinsic portion of the cascade is incomplete.

TISSUE FACTOR

Human tissue factor is a 43,000 dalton membrane glycoprotein that behaves as a receptor for factor VII and factor VIIa in the initiation of the extrinsic coagulation pathway. There are recent publications summarizing the purification, characterization and enzymology of tissue factor (Carson, 1987a; Nemerson, 1988). Molecular cloning of the cDNA of tissue factor has provided the amino acid sequence and other structural information relevant to its function in the coagulation cascade (Spicer, 1987; Morrisey, 1987). Figure 2 shows the first 219 amino acid residues that represent the extracellular part of the protein; it contains 3 N-linked carbohydrate binding sites, 5 half cystines for disulfide bonds and 3 tryptophan-lysine-serine tripeptides that may participate in the binding of factor VII/VIIa, factor X and factor IX. There is a hydrophobic 22 amino acid sequence that is the transmembrane portion of the protein and a 21 amino acid intracellular segment of the protein that may participate in some regulatory function of tissue factor activity. There is very little homology with either the vitamin K dependent serine proteinases that constitute the coagulation factors or other known proteins.

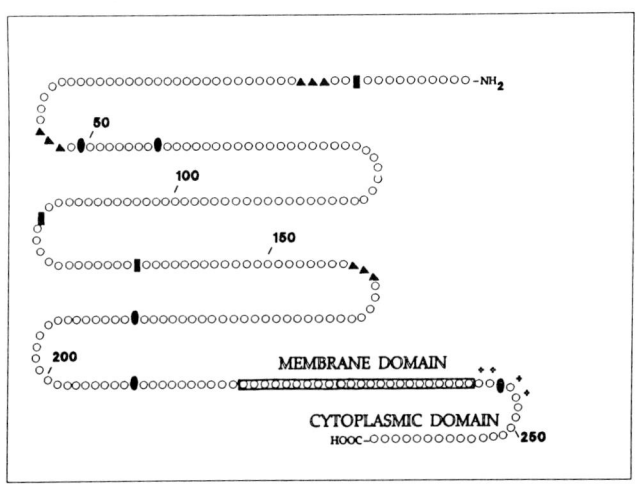

Figure 2

A Schematic Diagram of Tissue Factor. There are 3 N-linked carbohydrate attachment sites (▋), 5 ½-cystines (●) and 3 tryptophan-lysine-serine tripeptides (▲▲▲). It is a 263 amino acid polypeptide with a 219 amino acid extracellular segment, a 22 amino acid transmembrane segment and a 20 amino acid intracellular domain.

Since tissue factor is present on most normal and malignant cells, and most of these cells are not thrombogenic, the expression of procoagulant activity is probably tightly regulated. There are several mechanisms that participate in the regulation of tissue factor activity on the cell surface. Perturbation of the cell membrane is thought to facilitate the exposure of tissue factor to the extracellular environment and promote its procoagulant activity (Nemerson, 1982). Stimulation of monocytes with endotoxin and other substances promotes the synthesis of tissue factor and expression of its procoagulant activity (Rickles, 1983). There is a group of lipophilic substances found in plasma that affect tissue factor activity, including apolipoprotein A II and TFI (Carson, 1987b; Broze, 1987). Regulation of tissue factor activity may be associated with the metabolic modulation of the intracellular peptide by a mechanism not yet defined. Thus, the expression of tissue factor activity is regulated by cell membrane perturbation, factors that regulate the synthesis of the protein, extracellular inhibitors and probably intracellular metabolic events.

PROTHROMBINASE COMPLEX

The factor V/factor Xa reaction with prothrombin, referred to as the prothrombinase complex, is the subject of a recent review by Mann (1987). The rate of thrombin generation by the prothrombinase complex is 100,000 fold faster than by factor Xa in solution. The binding of factor V to a site (receptor) on the platelet facilitates this reaction; whether or not this site is a receptor protein or a unique phospholipid configuration is not known. Malignant cells appear to have the same or similar factor V binding properties (VanDeWater, 1985), such that they facilitate the assembly of the prothrombinase complex and the acceleration of thrombin production. Although it is not clear that acute leukemia cells have this factor V binding capacity, their close physical association with platelets and other cells in the blood (Tracy, 1985) should provide the appropriate ingredients for activity of the coagulation cascade. Thrombin activates the platelets, resulting in their participation in the thrombotic process and as well as their removal from the circulation.

CANCER PROCOAGULANT

The second procoagulant expressed by malignant cells, including acute non-lymphocytic leukemia cells, is cancer procoagulant (CP). CP is a 68,000 dalton cysteine proteinase that initiates coagulation by directly activating factor X in the coagulation cascade(Gordon, 1981a; Falanga, 1985). Until recently, CP was thought to be associated only with solid tumors (Gordon, 1979; Gordon, 1981b). Recently, peripheral blood and bone marrow cells from the 5 cytologic types of ANLL were studied to determine whether or not they contained cancer procoagulant. Procoagulant

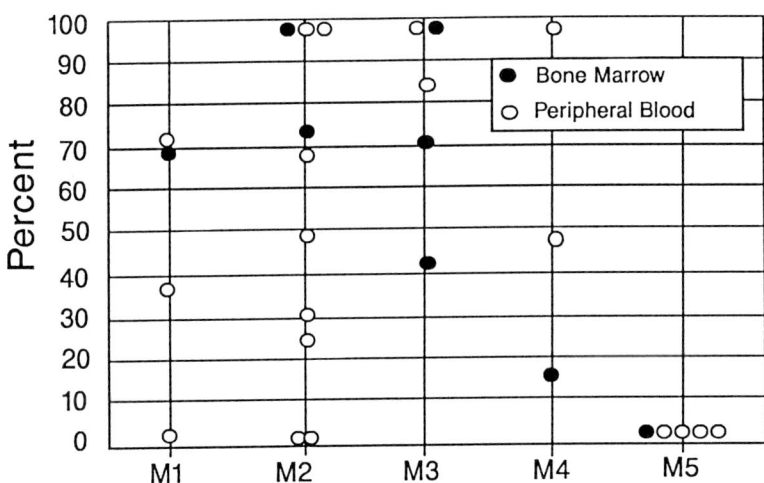

Figure 3.
The specific procoagulant activity of ANLL extracts in normal and factor VII deficient plasma was determined and the percent of the activity in the extracts from each cytologic subtype was calculated.

activity that initiated coagulation in the absence of factor VII was found in extracts of 4 of the 5 cytologic subtypes (Falanga, 1988). Factor VII independent activity ranged from 0 to 75% in the M1 subtype, 0 to 100% in the M2 subtype, 43 to 100% in the M3 subtype and 18 to 100 in the M4 subtype (Fig. 3). The M5 subtype had procoagulant activity similar to tissue factor of normal leukocytes. Thus, many of the extracts contained a significant portion factor VII independent activity.

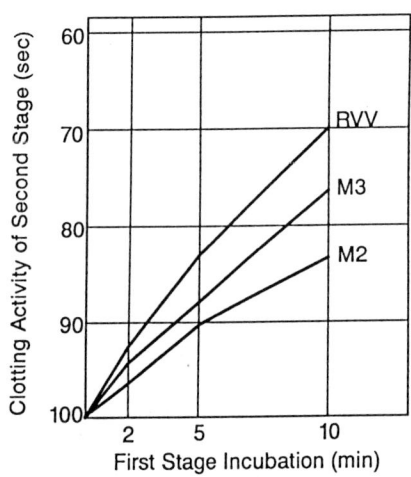

Figure 4. Pure factor X was incubated with pooled extracts from M2 and M3 ANLL cells and an RVV standard. Samples were removed at timed intervals and added to factor VII and X deficient plasma to assay the level of factor Xa produced in the first stage reaction mixture.

Figure 4 shows the ability of the procoagulant in pooled M2 and M3 extracts to directly activate pure bovine factor X in a two stage clotting assay. Russell's viper venom (RVV) a serine proteinase that is known to directly activate factor X, was used as a standard; the 2 extracts activated factor X in a similar fashion.

Pooled ANLL cell extracts were treated with either concanavalin A, to block tissue factor activity (Fig. 5), or iodoacetamide and $HgCl_2$, to block cysteine proteinase activity of cancer procoagulant

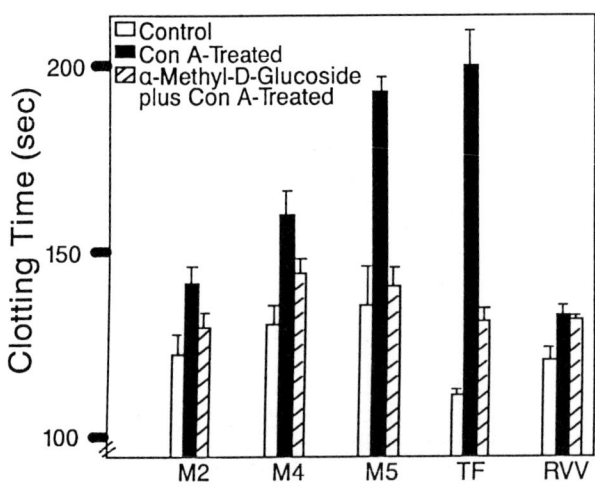

Figure 5. Con A or Con A and α-methyl glucoside was incubated with ANLL cell extracts or TF and RVV control and the loss of activity was compared to the untreated sample.

(Fig. 6), in an effort to further characterize the nature of the procoagulant activity in the extracts. The extract from the M5 subtype lost a comparable amount of activity as the tissue factor control while the M4 and M2 extract pools lost proportionally less activity, suggesting that the activity in the M4 and M2 extracts was composed of a smaller portion of tissue factor. In an analogous manner, the loss of activity of the pooled extracts after treatment with iodoacetamide and $HgCl_2$ shows that the activity of the M2 and M3 subtypes paralleled the loss of activity of the papain cysteine proteinase control. The loss of activity of the pooled M1 and M4 was less and the activity of the M5 subtype was comparable to the RVV serine proteinase control. Thus, the inhibition of procoagulant activity of the various subtypes was consistent with the expression of either tissue factor (M5) or CP (M3) or both tissue factor and CP (M1, M2, and M4).

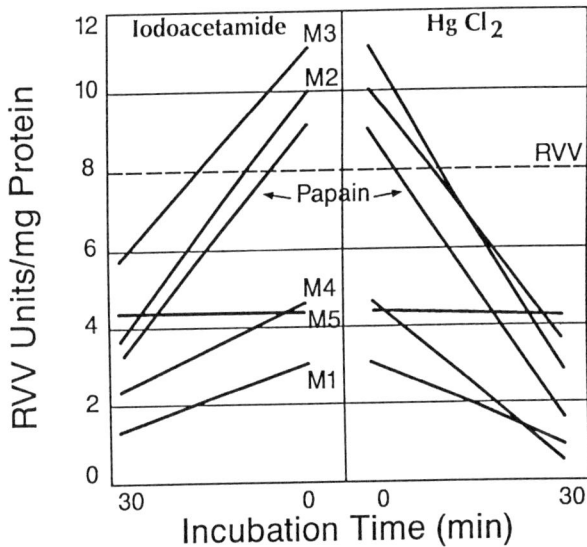

Figure 6. Iodoacetamide and $HgCl_2$ were incubated with either ANLL cell extracts or papain and RVV control procoagulants and the loss of activity was compared to the untreated sample.

DISCUSSION

There were two procoagulant activities in the ANLL cell extracts; they had the characteristics of both tissue factor and cancer procoagulant. It is not possible to quantitate the amount of these procoagulants in the cells because the method for cell extraction favors the recovery of cancer procoagulant while the recovery of tissue factor is not optimal. However, it is clear that the initiation of coagulation by these cells could proceed by either of two mechanisms, tissue factor or cancer procoagulant.

Several inhibitors of tissue factor activity are described above. There are probably comparable inhibitors of cancer procoagulant activity but they are not yet defined. Thus, it is not possible to determine the net procoagulant activity of malignant cells. It is the subject of current research efforts.

Figure 7 presents a schematic diagram summarizing the working hypothesis of procoagulants in acute non-lymphocytic leukemia. Tissue factor is a cell membrane receptor for factor VII that facilitates the activation of factor X and IX. Cancer procoagulant is released from the cells and can activate factor X. The net result of these activities is factor Xa which can bind to factor Va in the prothrombinase complex for the generation of thrombin. Thrombin converts fibrinogen to fibrin for polymerization by factor XIIIa as the final step in the coagulation cascade.

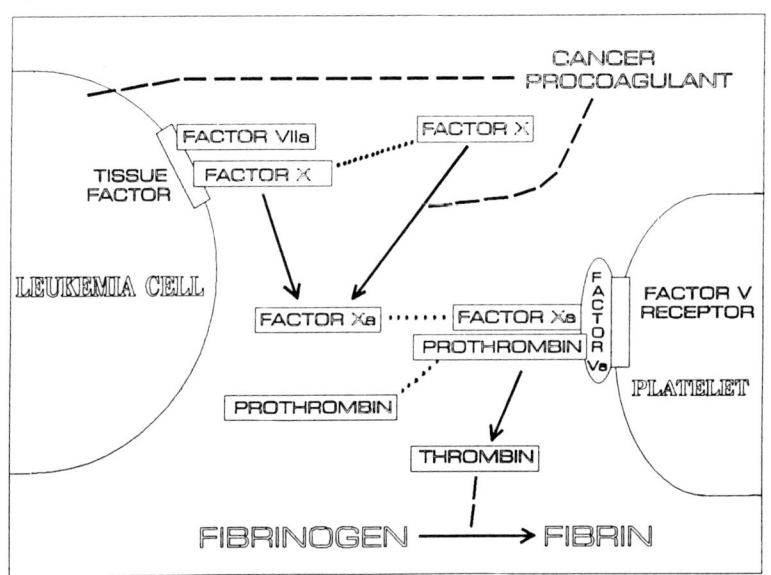

Figure 7.
A Schematic Diagram of Leukemia Cell Procoagulants. Cancer procoagulant and tissue factor-factor VIIa activate factor X. Factor V receptor on a platelet, binds factor Va; prothrombin and factor Xa assemble into the prothrombinase complex to produce thrombin. Thus, the leukemia cell, in concert with platelets, provides the necessary components to facilitate fibrin formation.

REFERENCES

Bauer, K.A. and Rosenberg, R.D. (1984): Thrombin generation in acute promyelocytic leukemia. Blood 64:791-796.

Berild, D., Hasselbalch, H. and Knudsen, J.B. (1987): Platelet survival, platelet factor-4 and bleeding time in myeloproliferative disorders. Scand.J Clin.Lab.Invest. 47:497-501.

Bratt, G., Blomback, M. and Lockner, D. (1985): Factors and inhibitors of blood coagulation and fibrinolysis in promyelocytic leukemia. Scand.J Clin.Lab.Invest.[Suppl] 178:81-83.

Bratt, G., Blomback, M., Paul, C., Schulman, S., Tornebohm, E. and Lockner, D.(1985): Factors and inhibitors of blood coagulation and fibrinolysis in acute nonlymphoblastic leukaemia. Scand.J Haematol. 34:332-339.

Broze, G.J. and Miletich, J.P. (1987): Isolation of a tissue factor inhibitor produced by HepG2 hepatoma cells. Proc. Natl. Acad. Sci. 84:1886-1890.

Carson, S.D. (1987): Tissue factor-initiated blood coagulation. Prog. Clin. Path. 9:1-14.

Carson, S.D. (1987): Tissue factor (coagulation factor III) inhibition by apolipoprotein A II. J. Biol. Chem. 262:718-721.

Egbring, R., Schmidt, W., Fuch, G. and Havemann, K. (1977): Demonstration of Granulocytic Proteases in Plasma of Patients with Acute Leukemia and Septicemia with Coagulation Defects. Blood 49:219-231.

Falanga, A. and Gordon, S.G. (1985): Isolation and characterization of cancer procoagulant: A cysteine proteinase from malignant tissue. Biochem. 24:5558-5567.

Falanga, A., Alessio, M.G., Donati, M.B. and Barbui, T. (1988): A new procoagulant in acute leukemia. Blood 71:870-875.

Gordon, S.G. (1981): A proteolytic procoagulant associated with malignant transformation. J. Histochem. & Cytochem. 29:457-463.

Gordon, S.G. and Cross, B.A. (1981): A Factor X Activating Cysteine Protease from Malignant Tissue. J. Clin. Invest. 67:1665-1671.

Gordon, S.G., Franks, J.J. and Lewis, B.J. (1979): Comparison of procoagulants from normal and malignant human tissue. J. Natl. Cancer Inst. 62:773-776.

Linman, J.W. and Bagby, G.C. (1978): The preleukemic syndrome (hemopoietic dysplasia) Cancer 42:854.

Mann, K.G. (1987): The assembly of blood clotting complexes on membranes. TIBS 12:229-233.

Marlar, R.A., Endres-Brooks, J. and Miller, C. (1985): Serial studies of protein C and its plasma inhibitor in patients with disseminated intravascular coagulation. Blood 66:59-63.

Morrissey, J.H., Fakhrai, H. and Edgington, T.S. (1987): Molecular cloning of the cDNA for tissue factor the cellular receptor for the initiation of the coagulation protease cascade. Cell 50:129-135.

Nemerson, Y. (1988): Tissue Factor and Hemostasis. Blood 71:1-8.

Nemerson, Y. and Bach, R. (1982): Tissue factor revisited. Prog. in Hemostasis and Thrombosis 6:237-261.

Rickles, F.R. and Edwards, R.L. (1983): Activation of blood coagulation in cancer: Trousseau's syndrome revisited. Blood 62:14-31.

Spicer, E.K., Horton, R., Bloem, L., Bach, R., Williams, K.R., Guha, A. Kraus, J. Lin, C. Nemerson, Y. and Konigsberg, W.H. (1987): Isolation of cDNA clones coding for human tissue factor: Primary structure of the protein and cDNA. Proc. Natl. Acad. Sci. 84:5148-5152.

Sterrenberg, L., Haak, H.L., Brommer, E.J.P. and Nieuwenhuizen, W. (1985): Evidence of Fibrinogen Breakdown by Leukocyte Enzymes in a Patient with Acute Promyelocytic Leukemia. Haemostasis 15:126-133.

Tracy, P.B., Eide, L.L. and Mann, K.G. (1985): Human prothrombinase complex assembly and function on isolated peripheral blood cell populations. J. Biol. Chem. 260:2119-2124.

VanDeWater, L., Tracy, P.B., Aronson, D., Mann, K.G. and Dvorak, H.F. (1985): Tumor cell generation of thrombin via functional prothrombinase complex. Cancer Res. 45:5521-5525.

RESUME

Patients with acute non-lymphocytic leukemia, particularly those with promyelocytic leukemia, frequently have of coagulation abnormalities ranging from bleeding to clotting. This discussion focuses on the initiation of coagulation by procoagulant factors as a likely cause for the activation of the coagulation cascade. This could lead to either clotting diathesis, if sufficient activation occurs, or bleeding diathesis, if a chronic low grade activation causes depletion of either clotting factors or inhibitors. The procoagulants that are participants in this process are tissue factor or cancer procoagulant. Tissue factor is a membrane factor VII receptor glycoprotein that is associated with all normal and malignant cells. Its amino acid sequence reveals a 219 external segment with 3 glycosylation sites, 4 half-cystines and 3 tryptophan-lysine-serine tripeptides that may bind factors VII, IX and X. There is a 23 amino acid transmembrane segment and a 22 amino acid intracellular segment that may participate in metabolic control of tissue factor activity. A factor V receptor on solid tumor cells and platelets may be associated with ANLL cells; it is responsible for accelerating the prothrombinase complex reaction. Cancer procoagulant was originally described associated with solid tumor cells but recent studies have demonstrated that it is also associated with ANLL cells. Either bone marrow or peripheral blood cells were extracted and the procoagulant activity was studied. Its activity in factor VII deficient plasma ranged from 0 to 100% in M1, M2, M3 cytologic subtypes; M4 had less and M5 had no factor VII independent activity. The M2 and M3 extracts directly activated factor X in a 2 stage clotting assay. The M1, M2 and M3 extracts were inhibited by iodoacetamide and $HgCl_2$ (cysteine proteinase inhibitors) while the M5 and, to a lesser extent, the M4 extracts were inhibited by concanavalin A (tissue factor inhibitor). Thus, ANLL cells have both tissue factor and cancer procoagulant for the initiation of coagulation.

Disappearance of cancer procoagulant (CP) from bone marrow of ANLL patients after complete remission induction

A. Falanga, M.G. Alessio*, R. Consonni, G. Colombi, M.B. Donati, T. Barbui

Divisione di Ematologia, Ospedali Riuniti di Bergamo, Istituto Mario Negri, Milano and Consorzio Mario Negri Sud, S. Maria Imbaro, Italy

ABSTRACT

The occurrence of severe acquired coagulopathy has been frequently reported in leukemic patients. Extracts of blast cells from patients with acute non lymphoid leukemia (ANLL) have been recently shown to possess a new procoagulant (Falanga et al., 1988) with characteristics of Cancer Procoagulant (CP), a Factor VII (FVII) independent, Factor X (FX) activating cysteine proteinase, described so far only in malignant tissue (Donati et al., 1986).
To verify whether CP activity is strictly associated with the presence of leukemic cells in bone marrow, nine ANLL patients, positive for CP in the acute phase of their desease, have been studied at different time intervals during induction and after achievement of complete remission (CR). Four of them showed a significant decrease ($p<0.05$) of F VII independent activity in an intermediate phase of partial remission. All of them showed a complete absence of this activity upon CR.
After an 18 months follow up, reappearance in two patients of a F VII independent activity, sensitive to cysteine proteinase inhibitors, was followed by morphologically documented bone marrow relapse.
These data suggest that CP detection may be a useful tool for revealing the presence of blast cells in ANLL.

Key words: Procoagulant Activity, Cancer Procoagulant (CP), Acute Non Lymphoid Leukemia (ANLL), Complete Remission (CR), Relapse.

This work was partially presented at the XXIX Congress of the American Society of Hematology, Washington, DC, 1987 and published in Abstract form in Blood (suppl. 1) 70: 199a, 1987
* Dr. M.G..Alessio is recipient of a fellwship of the Associazione Italiana per la Ricerca sul Cancro.

INTRODUCTION

A new procoagulant has been recently described in blast cells from different subtypes of ANLL. It shows characteristics consistent with those of CP, a cysteine proteinase that directly activates Factor X, independently from the presence of Factor VII. This activity is present in all ANLL morphologic subtypes but M5, and is significantly higher ($p<0.01$) in the M3 subgroup (Falanga et al.,1988).
To verify if CP activity is a property of leukemic cells and how early before relapse it can be detected in bone marrow, a group of ANLL patients has been repeatedly studied during and after CR induction. The results of this study are here presented.

PATIENTS AND METHODS

Nine patients with ANLL, 2 M1, 2 M2, 5 M3 (according to the FAB classification), 6 males and 3 females; age range 18-62 years, showing CP activity in bone marrow at diagnosis, have been studied upon achievement of CR. Eigth of them have been reanalyzed after CR at different time intervals over a period of about 20 months. Four of these patients have been also tested during an intermediate phase of partial remission before CR.
Blast cells were obtained from bone marrow (3-6 ml) and separated from granulocytes by Ficoll-Hypaque density gradient centrifugation. Extracts were made at 4° C for 3 hrs in 20 mM Veronal Buffer (pH 7.8). Protein contents were determined by Bradford's method (Bradford, 1976).
Procoagulant activity assay was performed by the one stage recalcification time of normal human plasma. Independence from coagulation F VII, a CP property, was tested by the ricalcification assay of F VII deficient plasma (Gordon & Cross, 1981). To determine the sensitivity to cysteine proteinase inhibitors, another characteristic of CP, samples were incubated for 30 min at room temperature with iodoacetamide (2 mM) or $HgCl_2$ (0.1mM) before the plasma recalcification tests. Russell's Viper Venom (RVV) and papain were used as a serine proteinase and a cysteine proteinase controls, respectively. Activity of samples was expressed as arbitrary units of RVV/mg protein.
The immunoreactivity of the extracts to a goat antiserum raised against purified CP (Falanga & Gordon, 1985) was tested by Ouchterlony immunodiffusion in agar gel.

RESULTS AND DISCUSSION

As shown in Table 1, blast extracts at diagnosis were able to express, like CP, a FVII independent procoagulant activity which ranged from 100.8 to 1.3 Units/mg prot. This activity was also significantly reduced ($p<0.01$) by treatment with inhibitors of cysteine proteinases (iodoacetamide, 2mM and $HgCl_2$, 0.1mM) and selected samples cross-reacted to a polyclonal anti-CP antibody (not shown).

Upon CR, a fall of such procoagulant to zero Units/mg prot was recorded and, in 3 out of 3 cases tested, no immuno-reactivity with an anti-CP antibody was observed.

The activity in the absence of Factor VII, measured in 4 patients (1 M1, 3 M3) during an intermediate phase of partial remission, decreased from mean value of 38.9 ± 24 Units/mg prot to mean value of 10.5 ± 6.29 Units/mg protein ($p<0.05$), suggesting a parallel reduction of both CP and tumor burden.

TABLE 1

Specific activity in normal plasma (NHP) and factor VII deficient (F VII-D) plasma of ANLL samples at diagnosis and upon complete remission.

Patient	ANLL TYPE	ANLL RVV Units/mg protein		COMPLETE REMISSION RVV Units/mg protein	
		NHP	FVII-D	NHP	FVII-D
1	M1	13.7	10.4	0	0
2	M1	21.2	1.5	6.6	0
3	M2	19.7	19.7	0	0
4	M2	16.8	12.7	0	0
5	M3	32.4	25.7	5	0
6	M3	100.8	100.8	0.6	0
7	M3	37.2	32.6	0	0
8	M3	5.9	1.3	0	0
9	M3	68.4	65.5	0	0

A 20 months follow up of 8 patients in CR (Table 2) revealed no F VII independent activity in all of them, except two (1 M1 and 1 M3). These latter showed, on the 18th month, an increase of specific activity from 0 to 13.7 Units/mg prot (patient M1) and from 0 to 4.87 Units/mg prot (patient M3).

TABLE 2
Relationship between expression of CP and presence of blasts in bone marrow.

	TIME (MONTHS)								
	0	1	2	//	18	21	22	22.5	23
Patient 1(M1)									
Activity in FVII-D Plasma (Units/mg prot)	10.4	n.t.*	0		13.7	8.4	0	n.t.	n.t.
Bone marrow blasts (%)	100	n.t.	0		75	25	0	n.t.	n.t.
Patient 5 (M3)									
Activity in FVII-D Plasma (Units/mg prot)	25.7	16.4	0		0.9	4.8	18.7	34.7	0
Bone marrow blasts (%)	100	50	0		0	20	100	100	0

* n.t. = not tested

A contemporary gradual increment of bone marrow leukemic blasts was documented. A new drop down to zero of procoagulant activity was associated with second remission.

These data suggest that CP activity is a property of leukemic cells. Its detection may be a useful tool for the diagnosis of early relapse in ANLL.

REFERENCES
Bradford, M.M. (1976). A rapid and sensitive method for the qualification of microgram quantities of protein utilizing the principle of dye-binding. Anal. Biochem. 72, 248-254.
Donati, M.B., Gambacorti-Passerini, C., Casali, B., Falanga, A., Vannotti, P., Fossati, G., Semeraro, N. and gordon, S.G. (1986) Cancer Procoagulant in Human Tumor Cells: Evidence from melanoma Patients. Cancer Res. 46, 6471-6474
Falanga, A. and Gordon, S.G. (1985). Isolation and characterization of cancer procoagulant : a cysteine proteinase from malignant tissue. Biochemistry 24, 5558-5567.
Falanga, A., Alessio, M.G., Donati, M.B., and Barbui, T. (1988) A New Procoagulant in Acute Leukemia. Blood 71, 870-875.
Gordon, S.G. and Cross, B.A. (1981). A Factor X activating cysteine protease from malignant tissue. J. Clin. Invest. 67, 1665-1671.

Cancer procoagulant activity as marker in a case of early cutaneous relapse of promyelocytic leukemia

L. Borin, C. Lanzafame, L. Baldicchi, G. Gambacorti Passerini, E. Pogliani, G. Corneo

Sezione di Ematologia, Ospedale San Gerardo, Monza and Istituto Nazionale dei Tumori, Milano, Italy

RESUME

Patients with acute leukemias have a high incidence of thromboembolic and/or hemorragic disorders.
We have studied six patients with M3 subtype of ANLL; they all showed high cancer procoagulant (CP) activity, which disappeared during remission.
In one of these cases, tissue extract made from a bone marrow biopsy during remission (blasts less than 5%) again expressed factor VII-independent activity (5U RVV/mg protein). At the same time the patient showed cutaneous nodules histologically defined "leukemidis". Tissue extract from cutaneous cells expressed CP activity (29.8 U RVV/mg protein), which was sensitive to cysteine proteinase inhibitors.
Cutaneous infiltration did not respond to chemiotherapic treatment and in tissue extract from bone marrow (blast less than 5%) there still was CP activity (9.10 U RVV/mg protein).

KEYWORDS
Acute promyelocytic leukemia, cancer procoagulant activity, thrombosis, hemorrhage

INTRODUCTION

Tissue extracts from leukemic cells of ANLL (acute non lymphoblastic leukemia) patients express a procoagulant activity (Falanga et al. 1988) This activity bears the enzymatic and immunologic characteristics of CP activity, a cysteine-proteinase which directly activates coagulation Factor X, and previously detected in tumor tissue from solid neoplasms. Particularly, cell extracts from promyelocytic leukemias are significantly more active than all other samples.

SUBJECTS AND METHODS
Patients
Eight patients, two males and six females (age range, 4 to 45 years) affected by ANLL, M3 subtype, have been studied. All patients have been evaluated at the onset of the disease and during their follow-up.

Cell extracts
Peripheral blood marrow samples were collected in 3.8% Na-citrate and diluted in phosphate-buffered saline, ph 7.4. Mononuclear cells were then isolated by Ficoll Hypaque (Limphoprep. Nyegaard, Oslo) density gradient centrifugation. After separation, the cells obtained were suspended in 20 mmol/L veronal buffer, ph 7,8 at the concentration of 50x10 cells/µl and preserved at 80°C.

Protein determination
Proteins were determined by Bradford's method.

Procoagulant activity assay
The procoagulant activity of extracts was tested by the one-stage plasma recalcification assay using a 202 A type clot timer (Heller Laboratories, Santa Rosa, California). Briefly, 0.1 ml sample was added to 0 1 ml plasma and prewarmed for one minute at 37°C; the reaction was started by adding 0.1 ml of 0.025 mol/L $CaCl_2$. The dependence on coagulation factor VII (FVII) was tested by using congenitally VII deficient plasma (Dade Division, Pharmaseal, Trieste, Italy).

Coagulation standard controls were tissue thromboplastin (rabbit brain thromboplastin; Sigma Chemical Co, St. Louis) and Russell's viper venom (RVV, X activating enzyme; Sigma).

The procoagulant activity of samples or standard controls was expressed as seconds or as the percent decrease in the clotting time compared with the corresponding buffer blank (blank time-sample clotting time/blank time).
The specific activity of samples was expressed as units of RVV per milligram-protein. Units were calculated on a standard curve prepared with different concentrations (from 10^{-1} to 10^{-6}) of RVV according to Gordon and Lewis (1978).

Inhibition studies
To determine whether the procoagulant activity of leukemic cell extracts was sensitive (like CP) to cysteine proteinase inhibitors, samples were preincubated for 30 minutes at 25°C with iodoacetamide (2mmol/L) or $HgCl_2$ (0.1mmol/L) before being used in the plasma recalcification test.

To assess whether the samples were sensitive (like TF) to the inhibitory effect of concanavalin A (Con A, Sigma), they were incubated with the inhibitor (100 µg/ml, final concentration) for one hour at 37°C and then assayed for procoagulant activity. Reversion of the Concanavalin A inhibition by α-metil-D-glucoside (Sigma) was also performed.

Skin biopsy
Punch biopsies obtained from leukemic skin localizations in patient P.A. were processed as previously described (Gambacorti Passerini C. et al, 1988). The cell suspension thus obtained was then processed in the same way as the other samples. As for the other samples the percent of tumor cells exceeded 90%.

Results
All extracts obtained by peripheral blood or bone marrow at diagnosis contained a procoagulant activity; this activity ranged between 4 and 50 RVVUnits/mg protein

(Table I) and was independent from the presence of factor VII.
$HgCl_2$ significantly inhibited this procoagulant activity.
The patients subsequently underwent induction therapy; bone marrow samples, taken during remission (blasts less than 5%), showed disappearance of the VII independent procoagulant (CPA).

Table I. Disappearance of Cancer Procoagulant from bone marrow of patients in complete remission.

Clinical case	CP ACTIVITY (U RVV/mg protein)	
	ONSET	COMPLETE REMISSION*
C.L.	4.37	0
L.A.	50	0
C.E	9.34	0
C.P.	4	0
P.A.	27.84	0
M.M.	30	0

* Complete remission: blasts less than 5% in bone marrow.

In patient P.A. the CPA at diagnosis was 27.84 U/mg. CPA then disappeared from bone marrow samples obtained in two separate occasions during remission, but a sample subsequently taken continued to contain less than 5% blasts.
Two weeks later the patient developed disseminated cutaneous nodules which were biopsied and proved to be cutaneous localisations of acute non lymphoblastic leukemia. "Fig. 1".
The tumor cells obtained from the skin lesions produced a CPA of 29.8 U/mg.
The bone marrow continued to contain less than 5% of blasts but remained CPA positive. "Fig. 2"

Discussion

These data confirm the presence in acute non lymphoblastic leukemia (ANLL) cells of a procoagulant activity, independent from the presence of factor VII and sensitive to $HgCl_2$. On this basis this activity can be considered as CP.
The levels of CP activity followed the course of the disease, disappearing from remission bone marrows.

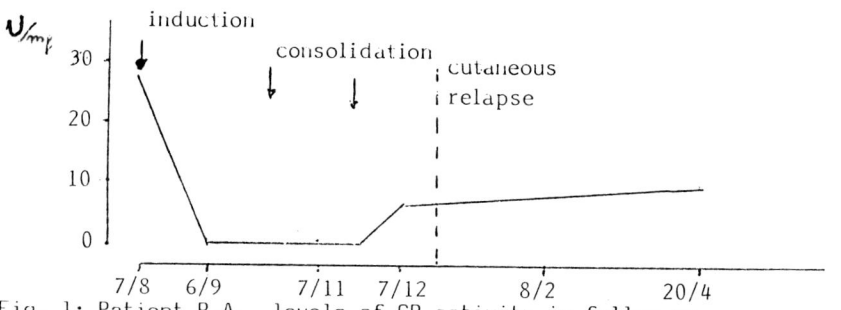

Fig. 1: Patient P.A., levels of CP activity in follow-up.

CP activity reappeared in a patient, although the bone marrow continued to be "in remission". Shortly after, this patient developed cutaneous leukemik relapses, which contained high levels of CP activity. These results, besides confirming the presence of CP activity in ANLL cells, raise the question of whether CP activity determination, on bone marrow samples, could be used during the follow -up of patients in order to detect relapses early.

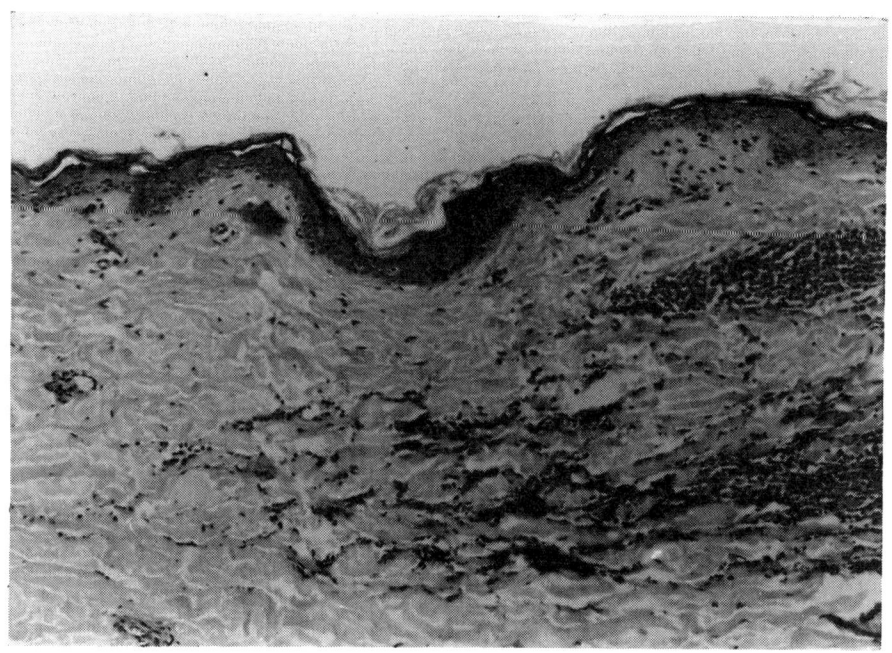

Fig 2 :Histological pattern of cutaneous localization

REFERENCES

Falanga A., Alessio M.G., Borin L., Pogliani E., Gugliotta L., Masera G., Donati M.B., Barbui T. (1987): Disappearance of cancer procoagulant (CP) from bone marrow of patients with acute non lymphoid leukemia (ANLL) in complete remission. Blood 70, Suppl. 1, 199a.

Falanga A., Alessio M.G., Donati M.B., Barbui T. (1988): A new procoagulant in acute leukemia. Blood 71, 870-875.

Gambacorti Passerini C., Raddrizani M., Erba E., Fossati G., Parmiani G. (1987): Lysis by activated lymphocytes of melanoma and small cell lung cancer cells surviving in vitro treatment with Mafosfamide. Cancer Res. 47, 2547-2552.

Gordon S.G., Lewis B.J. (1978): Comparison of procoagulant activity in tissue culture medium from normal and transformed fibroblasts. Cancer Res. 38, 2467.

Cancer procoagulant in acute lymphoid (ALL) and non lymphoid leukemia (ANLL)

A. Falanga, M.G. Alessio*, R. Consonni, G. Colombi, M.B. Donati, T. Barbui

Divisione di Ematologia, Ospedali Riuniti di Bergamo, Istituto Mario Negri, Milano and Consorzio Negri Sud, S. Maria Imbaro, Italy

ABSTRACT

Two procoagulant activities have been so far described in leukemic blasts: Tissue Factor (TF), a membrane glycoprotein, which activates coagulation in the presence of factor VII, and Cancer Procoagulant (CP), a cysteine proteinase which directly activates factor X, in the absence of factor VII.
CP has been characterized in different subtypes (from M1 to M5) of ANLL (Falanga et al.,1988). We have here studied whether or not CP is also expressed in ALL.
Extracts from blast cells of 15 freshly diagnosed patients with ALL have been tested for their procoagulant properties . Nine samples (60%) shortened the recalcification time of normal human plasma. Six samples (40%) did not possess any procoagulant activity.
CP was correctly identified in 5 out of the 9 active samples by testing two properties: 1. independence from factor VII in triggering blood coagulation and 2. sensitivity to cysteine proteinase inhibitors. CP specific activity of ALL patients was significantly lower than that of all of the ANLL groups previously studied, but M4.

Key words: Procoagulant activity, Acute non Lymphoid Leukemia (ANLL), Acute Lymphoid Leukemia (ALL), Cancer Procoagulant (CP), Cysteine proteinases.

INTRODUCTION

Hemostatic disorders associated with acute leukemia may be at least partially related to the procoagulant activity of leukemic cells. Besides Tissue Factor (TF), the well known procoagulant of both normal and malignant tissue, another procoagulant has been described in leukemic cells of ANLL (Falanga et al.,1988).

---
* Dr. M.G. Alessio is recipient of a fellowship of the Associazione Italiana per la Ricerca sul Cancro

This procoagulant shows characteristics of CP, a factor VII (F VII) independent, factor X (F X) activating cysteine proteinase.

We have here studied 15 patients with ALL in order to investigate whether blast cells from ALL are able to express CP as well as cells from ANLL and whether CP activity, if present, is quantitatively comparable to that of ANLL.

These results provide evidence that a procoagulant with CP characteristics may be present also in the lymphoid phenotype of acute leukemia, although its expression is less prominent than in the malignant myeloid lineage.

PATIENTS AND METHODS

Fifteen patients with ALL, 8 males and 7 females (age range 7-47 years), were studied at diagnosis, before starting chemotherapy. Leukemic cells were obtained either from pheripheral blood (10 samples) or from bone marrow (5 samples). After collection in 3.8% Na citrate, samples were diluted in PBS pH 7.4. Mononuclear blast cells ($\geq 50 \cdot 10^6$) were purified on a Ficoll-Hypaque density gradient and resuspended in 20 mM Veronal Buffer pH 7.4. Extracts were made by incubating fresh cells at 4° C in 3 changes of 20 mM Veronal Buffer, 2 hrs each; the three extracts were pooled and concentrated 1:2 to 1:6 times on a Centricon 30 ultrafiltration membrane (Amicon Co, MA). Protein contents were determined by the Bradford's method (Bradford, 1976).

The procoagulant activity was tested by the one stage clotting test (Gordon & Cross, 1981) of normal or F VII deficient plasma. Russell's Viper Venom (RVV), the standard activator of FX, and Rabbit Brain Thromboplastin (RBT) acted as a positive and negative controls, respectively, for the test in the absence of F VII. Activity of samples was expressed as seconds or as Units of RVV/mg protein (1 unit= activity of 1 mequiv./ml RVV in the single stage clotting assay).

The inhibition study was performed by incubating samples with two cysteine proteinase inhibitors (iodoacetamide, 2 mM and mercury chloride, 0.1 mM) for 30 min at 37 ° C. prior to the one stage clotting test (Falanga & Gordon, 1985). Papain, a cysteine proteinase, and RVV, a serine proteinase, were the standard controls of this test.

RESULTS AND DISCUSSION

Table 1 shows the procoagulant activity and the inhibition characteristics of ALL blast extracts and standard controls. Nine samples (Group 1 + Group 2) were able to shorten the recalcification time of normal human plasma (NHP), however only Group 1 (5 samples) showed activity in both normal and FVII deficient plasma (F VII-D). Six samples (Group 3) were negative in both types of assay. To verify the similarity of Group 1 procoagulant to CP, extracts were analyzed for their sensitivity to two cysteine proteinase inhibitors. Treatment with iodoacetamide (2 mM) or with $HgCl_2$ (0.1 mM) reduced the activity of 7% - 92% and of 4% - 82%, respectively.

TABLE 1
Procoagulant activity and inhibition characteristics of 15 ALL cell extracts and controls.

		SPECIFIC ACTIVITY (RVV Units/mg prot.)		% INHIBITION Iodoacetamide	$HgCl_2$
	n	NHP*	FVII*	(2 mM)	(0.1 mM)
ALL SAMPLES					
GROUP 1	5	0.43-20.5	0.02-2.47	7-92	4-82
GROUP 2	4	1.1-2.14	0	-	-
GROUP 3	6	0	0	-	-
CONTROLS					
RVV	4	10.2-8.9	10-8.1	0	0
RBT	4	14.5-13	0	0	0
PAPAIN	4	12-10.3	11.2-9	75-77	82-89

Results are expressed as a range.
* NHP=normal human plasma; **FVII-D = FVII deficient plasma

Procoagulant specific activity of Group 1 ALL has been compared (Table 2) with specific activities of all previously studied ANLL subtypes. Total activity, as measured in normal plasma, was not different than that of M1, M2, M4 and M5 ANLL subtypes, although it was significantly lower than that of M3. On the other hand, statistical comparison of F VII independent procoagulants showed that ALL Group 1 had significantly less activity than M1, M2 and M3, but not than M4. M5 was not compared because it does not possess F VII independent activity

TABLE 2
Comparison of total and FVII independent specific activity between ALL Group 1 and M1 to M5 ANLL subtypes.

	n	SPECIFIC ACTIVITY NHP	p*	SPECIFIC ACTIVITY FVII-D	p*
ALL Group 1	5	10.38±7.9		1.12±1	
ANLL M1	4	6.85±5.6	n.s.	4.47±4.38	p<0.05
" M2	9	9.70±7.0	n.s.	7.50±7.70	p<0.025
" M3	5	73.10±58.4	p<0.0005	65.30±44.2	p<0.02
" M4	3	2.40±0.68	n.s.	1.30±0.79	n.s.
" M5	5	3.40±2.50	n.s.	0	-

*ANLL subtypes vs ALL Group 1   Results are espressed as mean± S.D.

In summary, a comparative study of CP expression in ALL and ANLL patients demonstrates that 1) 40% of ALL samples do not possess any procoagulant activity, whereas only 8% were negative in the ANLL series, previously analyzed; 2) CP activity in ALL is lower than in all types of ANLL, but M4.
These data suggest that the lymphoid phenotype is associated with a reduced expression of CP in comparison to the myeloid phenotype. These findings could correlate with the minor incidence of thromboembolic disorders complicating the clinical course of ALL.

REFERENCES

Bradford, M.M. (1976). A rapid and sensitive method for the qualification of microgram quantities of protein utilizing the principle of dye-binding. Anal. Biochem. 72, 248-254.

Falanga, A. and Gordon, S.G. (1985). Isolation and characterization of cancer procoagulant : a cysteine proteinase from malignant tissue. Biochemistry 24, 5558-5567.

Falanga, A., Alessio, M.G., Donati, M.B., and Barbui, T. (1988) A New Procoagulant in Acute Leukemia. Blood 71, 870-875.

Gordon, S.G. and Cross, B.A. (1981). A Factor X activating cysteine protease from malignant tissue. J. Clin. Invest. 67, 1665-1671.

Treatment with differentiation agents modifies the expression of procoagulant activities of cultured cells from human leukemias and myelodysplastic syndromes

G. Gamba, L. Dezza, L. Ponchio, E. Ascari

Dipartimento di Medicina Interna e Terapia Medica, Sezione di Clinica Medica II, Università di Pavia, IRCCS Policlinico S. Matteo, Pavia, Italy

INTRODUCTION

Procoagulant activities (PCA) could be considered as marker of neoplastic transformation of bone marrow myeloid cells, as in other malignancies (Donati et al, 1984). On the other hand some substances with inhibitory effect on cell proliferation "in vitro", such as gamma interferon (IFN), retinoic acid (RA) and desferrioxamine (DFO) are known to induce differentiation of human leukemic cells to granulocyte (RA) and monocyte-like cells (IFN and DFO) (Koeffler, 1986, Kaplinsky et al, 1987, Dezza et al, 1988, Carlo Stella et al, 1988).
The aim of our investigation was to evaluate the PCA behaviour in human leukemic cells in relation to the expression of cytochemical and immunological markers of cell differentiation after treatment with the mentioned agents.

METHODS

Patients: 3 patients with LANL (M4, M5, M6) and 4 patients with untreated MDS (2 with RAEB-T and 2 with RAEB) were studied. The diagnosis of LANL and MDS was made according to the French-American-British classification (Bennet et al, 1985). The patient with M5 leukemia presented laboratory and clinical features of DIC.

Cell line: HL60 promyelocytic leukemia cells in exponential growth were used for the experiments.

In vitro cultures: 1×10^6/ml bone marrow cells after centrifugation on a Ficoll-Hypaque gradient (density 1077 g/ml) and 0.2×10^6/ml HL60 cells were cultured in suspension in RPMI 1640 plus 10% fetal calf serum in the presence or absence of 10-10^3 u/ml of recombinant gamma IFN (rHu IFN) (Biogen Research Corp), 10^{-6}M retinoic acid (RA) (Sigma Chemical Co, St Louis, USA), 10 uM/l desferrioxamine (DFO) (CIBA-Geigy Laboratories, Milan, Italy), 10^{-7}M 12-0-tetradecanoylphorbol-13-acetate (TPA) (Sigma) for 5 days.

Cell differentiation: cells were assessed for cytochemical and mmunological changes as described by Carlo Stella et al (1988).

PCA evaluation: PCA was measured as capacity to shortening recalcification time (RT) of normal plasma and of FVII, and FX deficient plasmas by the cell suspensions (1×10^6 cells/ml).

RESULTS

After 5 days of culture without inducers, all the cells tested expressed PCA, however higher activity was observed in M5 samples.
Cells treated with DFO (10uM/l), rHuIFN (10^3 u/ml), TPA (10^{-6}M) exhibited monocytic features as evaluated with cytochemical and immunological markers, while RA (10^{-6}M) treated cells showed myeloid differentiation.

In HL60 cells, TPA was able to generate highly active PCA; rHuIFN only at high concentration increased the PCA expression, while DFO and RA treatments seemed to reduce it (Fig.1).

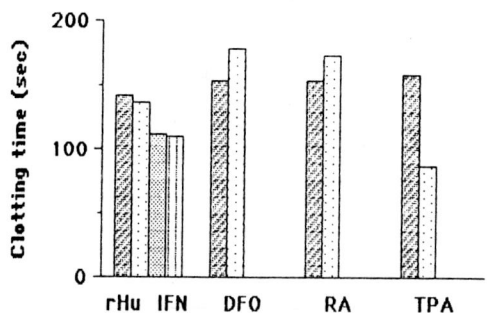

Fig. 1. Effect of various inducers on procoagulant activity of HL60 cells. Results are expressed as seconds normalized to a blank clotting time of 250 seconds.

untreated   treated (IFN 10 u/ml)   IFN 10^2 u/ml   IFN 10^3 u/ml

All samples of HL60 cell suspensions did not shorten the RT of FVII and FX deficient plasmas, showing TF type activity.
rHu IFN at low concentrations did not change or slightly reduced the PCA observed in untreated cells from leukemic and myelodysplastic patients, and, at higher concentrations, enhanced it.
DFO and RA had an inhibitory effect on PCA expressed by M4 and M5 cells, whereas in patients with MDS the PCA was differently affected by these agents (Tables I and II).

Table I. % decrease in Recalcification Time on normal, FVII and FX deficient plasmas induced by leukemic cells treated with the differentiation agents tested.

Cells (1x10⁶/ml)		Plasmas		
		Normal	F VII Deficient	FX Deficient
M4	untreated	48	60	0
	DFO	36	33	0
	rHuIFN 10 u/ml	40	62	0
	rHuIFN 10² u/ml	42	56	0
	rHuIFN 10³ u/ml	53	55	0
M5	untreated	60	10	0
	DFO	51	0	0
	RA	20	0	0
M6	untreated	58	22	0
	rHuIFN 10² u/ml	66	29	0
	rHuIFN 10³ u/ml	72	30	0

Table II. % decrease in Recalcification Time on normal, FVII and FX deficient plasmas induced by cells from myelodysplastic syndromes treated with the differentiation agents tested.

Cells (1x10⁶/ml)		Plasmas		
		Normal	F VII Deficient	FX Deficient
PD	untreated	55	5	0
	DFO	31	0	0
	RA	55	0	0
MR	untreated	42	8	0
	DFO	52	0	0
	RA	53	0	0
BB	untreated	34	18	0
	RA	8	33	0
	rHuIFN 10 u/ml	43	42	0
	rHuIFN 10² u/ml	43	34	0
	rHuIFN 10³ u/ml	53	28	0
LM	untreated	65	62	0
	RA	67	66	0
	rHuIFN 10² u/ml	71	60	0

Generally the cells presented a FVII and FX dependent PCA (TF-type), but some samples (M4, M6, BB, LM) showed also a partially independent FVII activity in promoting blood coagulation (CP-type).
Furthermore, the reduction of PCA expression observed in leukemic cells after treatments seemed to affect both FVII independent and dependent PCA.

DISCUSSION

Our study confirms that HL60 cells express cytochemical and immunologic characteristics typical of monocytes, after treatment with rHu IFN and DFO, and of granulocytes after treatment with RA, in agreement with other Authors, (Koeffler 1986, Kaplinsky et al 1987).
Furthermore, HL60 cells incubated with TPA were able to differentiate to monocyte-like cells and to increase their TF activity as observed also by Kornberg et al (1983). The increased PCA expression by the cells from leukemic and MDS patients, after rHu IFN treatment, may be attributed or to activation of monocytes contaminating the bone marrow samples, or to differentiation of blasts cells to activated monocytes, as it was the case for HL60 cells, and in agreement with the data reported by Carlo Stella et al (1988) in ANLL and MDS. On the other hand, the reduction of both TF-type and CP-type activities in leukemic cells after incubation with DFO and RA supports the existence of significant correlations between PCA expression and cell differentiation. In conclusion our data may indicate that the therapy with DFO and RA can be helpful not only to induce the leukemic blast cells to differentiate, but also to reduce the haemorragic complications due to the PCA produced by the leukemic cells.

REFERENCES

Bennet, J.M., Catowsky, D., Daniel, M.T., Flandrin, G., Galton, D.A.G., Granlick, H., Sultan, G. (1985): Proposed revised criteria for the classification of acute myeloid leukemia. Ann. Int. Med. 103,626-9.
Bross, K.J., Pangalis, G.A., Staatz, C.G., Blume, K.G. (1978): Demonstration of cell surface antigens and their antibodies by peroxidase-antiperoxidase method. Transplantation 25: 331-35.
Carlo Stella, C., Cazzola, M., Ganser, A., Bergamaschi, G., Meloni, F., Pedrazzoli, P., Bernasconi, P., Invernizzi, R., Hoelzer, D., Ascari, E. (1988): Recombinant gamma-interferon induces in vitro monocytic differentiation of blast cells from patients with acute nonlymphocytic leukemia and myelodysplastic syndromes. Leukemia 2,55-9.
Dezza, L., Cazzola, M., Danova, M., Carlo Stella, C., Bergamaschi, G., Brugnatelli, S., Invernizzi, R., Mazzini, G., Riccardi, A., Ascari, E. (1988): Effects of desferrioxamine on normal and leukemic human hematopoietic growth: in vitro and in vivo studies (submitted to Leukemia).
Donati, M.B., Semeraro, N., Gordon, S.G. (1984): Relationship between procoagulant activity and metastatic capacity of tumor cells. In K.V. Honn and B.F. Sloane (eds). Hemostatic mechanisms and metastasis. Boston: Martinus Nijhoff, 84-95.
Kaplinsky, C., Estrov, Z., Freedman, M.H., Gelfand, E.W., Cohen, A. (1987): Effect of deferoxamine on DNA synthesis, DNA repair, cell proliferation and differentiation on HL60 cells. Leukemia 1, 437-41.
Koeffler, H.P. (1986): Human acute myeloid leukemia lines: models of leukemogenesis. Sem. Hematol. 23,223-36.
Kornberg, A., Treves, A., Rachmilewitz, E.A., Fibach, E. (1983): Generation of procoagulant activity (PCA) by macrophage-like cells derived from acute and chronic myeloid leukemia cells in response to phorbol esters. Scan. J. Haematol. 31, 102-108.

ABSTRACT

We evaluated the expression of PCA in human promyelocytic cell line HL60 and in bone marrow mononuclear cells obtained from patients with acute leukemias (M4, M5, M6) and myelodysplastic syndromes, after 5 days of culture with rHu IFN ($10-10^3$ u/ml), RA (10^{-6}M) and DFO (10 uM/l). HL60 cells expressed PCA (TF-type), which were enhanced by treatment with rHu IFN at high concentration (10^3 u/ml) and reduced after exposition to RA and DFO. Leukemic cells were able to shorten RT of normal plasma. The RT reduction was more evident in untreated samples than after incubation with RA, DFO, whereas rHu IFN increased PCA expression also in fresh leukemic cells.

Disseminated intravascular coagulation in acute leukemia

F. Rodeghiero, G. Castaman

Department of Hematology and Hemophilia and Thrombosis Center, San Bortolo Hospital, 36100 Vicenza, Italy

ABSTRACT

A large body of evidence suggests that intravascular thrombin generation is a real event in acute leukemia complicated by clotting abnormalities. Indeed, these abnormalities can be accurately predicted by assuming thrombin generation and, moreover, specific thrombin markers have been clearly demonstrated in circulating blood of these patients. The trigger mechanism is thought to consist in the release of procoagulant material from blast cells. The attempts to further characterize these substances have been reviewed together with the prognostic significance of clotting abnormalities and the therapeutic possibilities to control bleeding in these patients.

KEY WORDS

Acute leukemia - Acute promyelocytic leukemia - Disseminated intravascular coagulation - Procoagulant activities - Heparin.

INTRODUCTION

Studies of blood coagulation in acute leukemia date back of several decades but literature survey shows a renewed and increased interest during the early sixties. At this time, the concept of excessive consumption of some blood coagulation factors as secondary to intravascular thrombin generation, triggered by the release into the bloodstream of thromboplastic substances, was rather new (Verstrate et al., 1965). Although this pathogenetic mechanism was not conclusively established, apart perhaps from some cases of coagulopathy secondary to obstetric complications, the concept of disseminated intravascular coagulation (DIC), as cause of multiple clotting deficiencies, become to be increasingly applied to a variety of clinical circumstances, including acute leukemia (AL). Other possible mechanisms such as iperactive fibrinolysis and release of proteolytic substances from blast cells, which also could be primarily involved, were the subject of limited investigation and, although often referred to as thoretical possibilities, were never conclusively investigated. These uncertainties are well reflected in a paper of Brakman and coworkers (1970) examining coagulation and fibrinolysis in AL. In this study one can find selected references to these early reports.

During the last two decades several studies have attempted to clarify the pathogenetic mechanism of coagulopathy in AL. These studies followed two principal lines of investigation. One aimed at characterizing the procoagulant as well as the fibrinolytic and proteolytic substances of leukemic cells. The other aimed at delucidating the pathogenetic mechanism of the hemostatic changes observed in circulating blood. After a brief account on the definition of this syndrome and its incidence, we shall review these studies together with clinical investigations concerning the prognostic significance and therapeutic management of clotting abnormalities in AL.

DEFINITION

There are no universally accepted minimal criteria for the diagnosis of DIC. It should be born in mind that test results may be influenced by the underlying disease (for example thrombocytopenia is not evaluable as a diagnostic criteria for DIC in AL) and by the synthetic liver capability. Laboratory tests currently used to diagnose DIC in AL include: fibrinogen; fibrinogen-fibrin degradation products (FDP); thrombin and prothrombin time; ethanol and protamine gelation tests. A diagnosis of DIC is usually done in presence of multiple abnormalities of the above mentioned tests. Minimal requirement for diagnosis are represented by the occurrence of hypofibrinogenemia (less than 130 to 150 mg%) or of increased FDP in serum (> 20 µg/ml) with the concomitant abnormality of at least one of the remaining tests. The term DIC in this report is used in the context of this definition. It is evident that this is a merely operational definition without the possibility of determining the pathogenetic mechanism of the coagulopathy in the individual patient. Indeed other mechanism, apart from intravascular clotting, could promote similar laboratory abnormalities (Merskey, 1973).

INCIDENCE AND CLINICAL SYMPTOMS

Apart from studies concerning acute promyelocytic leukemia (APL), almost invariably associated with DIC, scarce information is available on the incidence of this syndrome among the different types and subtypes of AL. On review of literature published from 1970 (when FDP assay became widely available to clinical laboratories), we were not able to find any prospective investigation on the incidence of DIC in acute lymphoblastic leukemia (ALL). Several clinical reports concerning patients with ALL and severe decompensated DIC complicated by hemorrhage have been published, totalizing to 16 described patients (table 1).

Table 1. Cases of ALL with decompensated DIC

Case	age/sex	phenotype	blasts/µl		Reference
1	27/M	T-ALL	73,950	A	Chorba et al. (1985)
2	52/M	NON-T	362,400	B	Guarini et al. (1980)
3	15/M	NON-T	1,600	B	Guarini et al. (1980)
4	30/M	NON-T	800	A	Guarini et al. (1980)
5	61/F	NON-T (Ph+)	26,200	B	Guarini et al. (1980)
6	9/F	NON-T	128,000	B	Champion et al. (1978)
7	13/M	NON-T	20,000	B*	Champion et al. (1978)
8	6/M	T-ALL	370,000	B	Champion et al. (1978)
9	6/-	ND	-	-	Gralnick et al. (1972)
10	18/-	ND	-	-	Gralnick et al. (1972)
11	12/-	ND	-	-	Gralnick et al. (1972)
12	15/-	ND	-	-	Gralnick et al. (1972)
13	3.5/-	ND	-	-	Gralnick et al. (1972)
14	17/F	ND	-	-	Niemetz & Nossel (1969)
15	0.1/F	NON-T	-	-	Bastard et al. (1985)
16	44/M	B-ALL	0	B	Daly et al. (1986)

A= DIC present at diagnosis; B= DIC after starting chemotherapy.
*= DIC developing during treatment for relapse.

In some cases DIC developed during rapid tumor cell lysis. No apparent relationship with T or B lineage or blast cell count exists. Mean fibrinogen was significantly lower and FDP significantly higher in patients with T-ALL in comparison with non-T ALL suggesting low grade DIC in T-ALL, however T-ALL cases were usually complicated by liver failure (French & Lilleyman, 1979). Higher incidence of hypofibrinogenemia in T-ALL not associated with overt DIC was also reported by Wada et al.(1982). The relative incidence of DIC to non-DIC cases is stated only in a paper of Guarini et al (1980) who found 4 cases of acute hemorrhagic defibrination (occurring after chemotherapy in 2 cases) among 52 adults with ALL. A similar incidence (6%) was found on review of 49 unselected cases of ALL, followed at our institution. In these cases the diagnosis was based on the above mentioned laboratory tests, independently from clinical severity (table 2).

Table 2. Incidence of DIC in the different types and subtypes of AL
(Hematology Department, Vicenza)

---

112 unselected cases of AML excluding APL since 1985

M1	4/26	15%
M2	6/37	16%
M4	4/26	15%
M5	4/19	21%
M6	1/4	25%
Overall	19/112	17%

62 unselected cases of APL (1970-87)

53/62   85%

49 unselected cases of ALL since 1985

3/49   6%

Close scrutinity of the recently published series (Al-Mondhiry, 1975; Sielgal et al., 1978; Spero et al., 1980), collecting data from unselected patients followed at specialized centers, shows 54 cases of DIC in AL out of 553 cases with DIC due to other causes. The ratio of ALL/ANLL among these 54 cases was 7/47 (14%). Of the 47 cases of DIC in ANLL 10 were in patients with APL. The overall incidence of DIC in ANLL is not known but, as suggested by the above cited studies and in keeping with clinical impression, is probably fairly higher than in ALL, even without considering cases of APL which represents no more than 5% of all cases of AL.

No data are available in the literature on the different incidence of DIC in the different subtypes of ANLL, classified according to FAB formulation (Bennet et al, 1976b). An overall incidence of 17% of DIC was found on review of 112 unselected cases with AL, excluding cases with APL, followed at our institution; no differences were observed among the different subtypes (table 2).

The close association of APL with severe hemorrhagic manifestations was already well identified by Hillestad in 1957. DIC as the cause of the derangement of coagulation observed in APL was recognized since the early sixties (Verstrate et al., 1965; Bernard et al., 1959; Didisheim et al., 1964) and in 1964 Baker et al. described a patient with APL and a typical clinical and laboratory picture of DIC in whom DIC was completely corrected by heparin administration. APL rapidly emerged as a unique form of acute myelogenous leukemia costantly associated with DIC and almost invariably presenting with hemorrhagic symptoms (Gralnick & Sultan, 1975). Hemorrhagic symptoms usually include petechiae, ecchymoses, hematuria, bleeding from venipuncture or more rarely from bone marrow sites. Epistaxis and gingival bleeding are frequent and menorrhagia, sometimes requiring massive transfusion, is very common in the menstruating age group. Cerebral hemorrhage may develop in a matter a few minutes or hours and be cause of death before any chemotherapy can be administered. Massive gastrointestinal bleeding is a second recognized cause of death in these patients. Usually bleeding symptoms precede diagnosis by 2-8 weeks (Gralnick & Sultan, 1975). These hemorrhagic manifestations are not accounted for by the degree of thrombocytopenia. DIC and hemorrhagic manifestation occurs, with a similar frequency, also in the recently identified microgranular variant of APL (Golomb et sl., 1980). However, although hemorrhagic phenomena predominate, venous as well as thromboembolic complications may occur in up to 2-5% of patients with APL as documented by a careful review of literature done by Groopman and Ellman (1979). Thrombotic symptoms were more rare in other types of AL. Fibrin thrombi have been recognized at autopsy in kidney, lung, adrenal, heart, liver and spleen in approximately 25% of cases (Groopman and Ellman, 1979). These findings have been recently confirmed by Tanaka and Imamura (1983) who have found presence of microthrombi in the vessels of at least three different organs in 16% of autopsied cases of APL.

Although costantly reported associated with DIC in early series, more recently published studies show that DIC is not invariably present in APL at diagnosis. In our clinical series the incidence was 85% (table 2), but a rate ranging from 60 to 95% has been reported (table 3). Moreover, surprisingly, sequential studies seem to suggest no higher incidence of DIC during chemotherapy (table 3).

Table 3. Prevalence of DIC in various series of APL

Pts/DIC	Diagnosis	After chemotherapy	NS	Reference
111/82	-	-	*	Marty et al. (1984)
24/22	22/18	24/22	-	Drapkin et al. (1978)
57/36	-	-	*	Cordonnier et al. (1985)
27/23	-	-	*	Goldberg et al. (1987)
16/16	16/12	16/16	-	Arlin et al. (1984)
57/47	57/39	57/47	-	Kantarjian et al. (1986)
62/52	62/52	-	-	Petti et al. (1987)
34/23	34/23	-	-	Sanz et al. (1988)
114/68	114/68	112/49	-	Hoyle et al. (1988)
24/23	-	-	*	McKenna et al. (1982)
526/391 (74%)	305/212 (69%)	209/134 (66%)		

NS= not stated; DIC diagnosed according to authors' criteria

However, since a close monitoring of the patients has not been carried out in all studies, short-lived DIC could have been overlooked. In our experience, in keeping with other authors (Gralnick et al., 1972, Gralnick and Sultan, 1975), the starting of inductive therapy usually is associated with a temporary worsening od DIC parameters, showing that probably tumor cell lysis is able to induce increased consumption of clotting components (see table 8).

PROCOAGULANT, FIBRINOLYTIC AND PROTEOLYTIC ACTIVITIES OF LEUKEMIC CELLS.

Coagulation abnormalities observed in the blood of leukemic patients are thought to be the product of changes induced on circulating substrates by clot-promoting, fibrinolytic or proteolytic activities released into circulation from leukemic cells.

At least three procoagulant activities (PA) have been described in tumor cells: tissue factor (TF), a glyco-lipoprotein that requires factor VII to activate coagulation factor X (Dvorak et al., 1983); Cancer procoagulant (CP), a cysteine proteinase which directly activates factor X (Gordon & Cross, 1981); the ability of certain specific membrane structures to facilitate the assembly of the prothrombinase complex (activated factor X and V in presence of calcium jons) (Vandewater et al., 1985). Whereas CP seems a specific tumor marker, having been found so far only in tumor cells and in human amnion-chorion tissue (Falanga & Gordon, 1985; Gordon et al., 1985; Donati et al., 1986), the two other activities are present in high activity in most of normal tissues. Prothrombinase assembly activity, however, has not been tested in leukemic cells. PA has been described in leukemic cells since 1954 (Eiseman & Stefanini, 1954). In 1967, Quigley firstly demonstrated thromboplastin activity in leukemic promyelocytes. Gralnick & Abrell (1973) studied the promyelocytes (both intact and after disruption) of few patients with APL and could demonstrate that APL cells, compared to normal polymorphonuclear cells and leukemic myeloblasts, consistently shortened the recalcification time (and partial thromboplastin time) of normal, as well as factor VIII and IX deficient plasma, but had no effect on factor X or X-VII deficient plasma. Although CP itself could influence these tests, the specific nature of this PA was functionally identified as tissue factor in a two-stage assay saturated with factor VII and X, in which the initial rate of factor X activation is measured and tissue factor is the rate limiting factor (Gralnick & Abrell, 1973). The increased TF activity was associated primarily with the granular and nuclear fractions with no activity in the supernatants. Subsequently Gouault-Heilmann et al (1975) demonstrated immunological cross-reactivity between human brain TF and the procoagulant factor isolated from leukemic promyelocytes; most of the TF activity of promyelocytes could be neutralized by anti-TF antibodies.

Several studies have attempted to correlate the presence of TF activity with a particular subtype of blast cell and the presence of DIC in the patient from whom the cells were obtained; PA was studied mainly in lysates, but in some cases also in intact cells. The high content of TF activity in leukemic promyelocytes was consistently confirmed in all studies (Sakuragawa et al., 1976; Wada et al., 1982; Guarini et al., 1985; Guarini et al., 1987), but high TF was found also in some cases of AML or exceptionally in ALL, especially of T-lineage (Wada et al., 1982). Leukemic promyelocytes possess high basal TF activity (Wada et al., 1982; Gralnick & Abrell, 1973; Sakuragawa et al., 1976; Guarini et al., 1985; Guarini et al., 1987), whereas this activity is usually greatly increased only after endotoxin stimulation in leukemic cells of monocytic origin (M4 and M5 FAB subtypes), even when basally low. This pattern seems to represent a distinctive feature of leukemic monocytic cells, similar to that of normal monocytes (Guarini et al., 1987). However, other studies do not support this conclusion, since monoblasts were found not to be able to produce PA after stimulation (Lyberg et al., 1983; Pogliani et al., 1986). A good correlation has been found between high TF activity and the presence of DIC in the patients from whom cells were harvested (Wada et al., 1982; Guarini et al., 1985). The ability to produce PA seems restrict to leukemic cell, whereas normal myeloid precursor cells, apart from monocytes, do not possess or produce PA (Guarini et al., 1986).

Recently, Falanga et al. (1988) were able to demonstrate CP activity in leukemic cells of myeloid lineage, especially in the M3 subgroup, but not in any of 9 cell-preparations from patients with M4 or M5 leukemia. In all subtypes (M1 to M5) some TF activity, especially high in M2 and M3 cases, was also found and could be separated from CP. Since both activities contribute to the shortening of the recalcification time, it is possible that in early studies the combined effect of both these activities has been attributed to TF.

Fibrinolytic and proteolytic activity of leukemic cells was the subject of limited investigation. Gralnick and Abrell (1973) studied fibrinolytic activity of blasts from APL and other AML on fibrin plates (with and without plasminogen) and proteolytic activity on casein or denaturated hemoglobin, both at acid and physiological pH. These authors showed that leukemic promyelocytes (3 out of 4 preparations) possessed high fibrinolytic activity (not linked to increased plasminogen activator), but not parallel to the greatly increased TF activity. Proteolytic activity was also slightly increased in 3 of the preparations. Wilson et al. (1983) demonstrated that peripheral blasts from patients with ANLL were able to secrete tissue-type and urokinase-type plasminogen activators; the amount of plasminogen activator secreted was not correlated with the clinical severity of the disease.

Human granulocytes are known to contain two proteolytic enzymes, which in high concentrations are capable of degrading coagulation factors, namely elastase-like protease (ELP) and chymotrypsin-like protease (CLP) (Schmidt et al., 1974). These enzymes are present in normal myeloid cells after the stage of myeloblast and are contained in the primary azurophilic granules (Dewald et al., 1975) and, by inference, they are thought to be contained also in the granules of some myeloid blasts. Although never isolated from leukemic cells and only histochemically detected, their release into circulation in some cases of acute leukemia has been inferred from the detection of increased amount of complexes of ELP and CLP with their main plasma inhibitor, namely α-1-antitrypsin (Egbring et al., 1977).

CLOTTING ABNORMALITIES AND ITS PATHOGENETIC MECHANISM

If intravascular generation of thrombin is indeed the key event in the pathogenesis of clotting abnormalities in AL, a complex array of changes can be predicted to occur on clotting substrates. In turn, the demonstration of these changes in circulating blood of patients with AL can be used to prove the hypotesis of thrombin generation as the main cause of these hemostatic abnormalities.

The sequence of pathophysiological events, which can be anticipated to occur on the basis of thrombin intravascular generation, can be schematically summarized in the following steps.

Step 1: The release of procoagulants from blast cells activates clotting system with generation of thrombin from its parental molecule prothrombin by the release of prothrombin activation fragments F1+2.

Step 2: Thrombin activates factor V and VIII and subunit A of factor XIII.

Step 3: Thrombin causes the selective release of a small N-terminal peptide (fibrinopeptide A, FPA) from fibrinogen. After FPA release, fibrinogen polymerizes into fibrin and fibrin undergoes cross-linking by activated subunit A of factor XIII.

Step 4: Thrombin is neutralized by its specific inhibitor antithrombin III (AT-III) by the formation of 1:1 stoichiometric AT-III/thrombin complexes. Protein C is also possibly activated by thrombin in presence of thrombomodulin - a cofactor of the reaction present on endothelial cell surface - and activated protein C inactivates factor V and VIII.

Step 5: Coagulation activation causes secondary activation of fibrinolytic system, with the subsequent conversion of plasminogen into plasmin, and digestion of cross-linked fibrin with generation of cross-linked FDP. Plasmin is specifically neutralized by α-2-antiplasmin.

Specific clotting abnormalities found in AL can be attributed to each of these steps.

Step 1: High levels of prothrombin activation fragments, as detected by a specific developed radioimmunoassay, have been demonstrated by Bauer and Rosenberg (1984) in patients with APL.

Step 2: Normal or even shortened APTT is often observed during DIC in AL. This reflects the continuous activation of factor VIII, as also suggested by the presence of high levels of this factor obtained using one stage methods, sensitive to activated factor. Rarely, APTT becomes prolonged in patients with decompensated DIC. Prothrombin time is almost invariably prolonged due to the thrombin-dependent consumption of factor V, considered a prognostic negative factor by some authors, and also of factor II. In patients with DIC, subunit A and B of factor XIII are very low (Egbring et al, 1977; Rodeghiero et al, 1980, 1981, 1984a), clearly suggesting thrombin generation since subunit A is sensitive to thrombin but completely insensitive to plasmin. The concomitant reduction of thrombin-resistant subunit B is also consistently observed. This has been interpreted by Egbring et al (1977) as an evidence against thrombin activation of factor XIII and this finding has been used to support the hypothesis of proteolytic degradation. However, the reduction of subunit B may well be due to a homeostatic mechanism, which has been shown to be operating in congenital factor XIII deficiency (Rodeghiero et al, 1981).

Step 3: Increased FPA levels (Myers et al, 1981; Gugliotta et al, 1984; Rodeghiero et al, 1988) have been demonstrated in patients with AL, especially in APL subtype (Bauer and Rosenberg, 1984; Rodeghiero et al, 1988). Moreover, the observation of high urinary FPA levels during 24 hours demonstrate that fibrin formation is an ongoing process (Rodeghiero et al, 1988). The presence of decreased fibrinogen level associated with a shortened fibrinogen survival have been recognized since early '70 (Givelber & Gralnick, 1972; Al-Mondhiry et al., 1975; Barbui et al., 1976). Using FPA turnover as a marker of thrombin-dependent catabolic fraction of fibrinogen, we and other demonstrated that about 50% of fibrinogen is catabolized by thrombin in patients with AL and DIC, whereas patients without DIC showed a thrombin-dependent catabolism similar to that observed in normal volunteers (table 4; Yoda & Abe, 1981).

Table 4. ^{125}I-Fibrinogen survival in acute leukemia with and without DIC

	NORMAL	AL WITH DIC (4 cases)	AL WITHOUT DIC (9 cases)
Thrombin-dependent catabolic fraction (%)	5-10	48 (13)*	10 (6)
Fibrinogen survival T 1/2 (days)	4.2 (0.3)	0.6 (0.1)§	1.1 (0.2)§#

* P < 0.01 versus normal and AL without DIC
§ P < 0.01 versus normal
# P < 0.05 versus Al with DIC

Step 4: Increased levels of AT III-Thrombin complexes have been detected when measured with sensitive techniques (Bauer and Rosenberg, 1984; Avvisati et al, 1988) but not employing crossed immunoelectrophoresis (Rodeghiero & Barbui, 1977). Slightly decreased AT III concentration (Sandler et al, 1983; Rodeghiero et al, 1984b) has been observed in AL. The fact that AT III is only slightly reduced in DIC is well understandable if one condiders that the stoichiometry of the reaction is exceedingly in favour of AT III, present in a large excess, on a molar basis, in comparison to thrombin. In keeping with this, Muller-Berghaus et al (1985) demonstrated that in rabbits infused with large amount of thrombin AT III level remained almost unchanged despite severe defibrination. Moreover, we have clearly demonstrated that liver function is the main determinant of AT III concentration in AL.

As in the case of AT III, also protein C is only slightly reduced in AL with DIC (Rodeghiero et al, 1984; Mimuro et al, 1987; Avvisati et al, 1988). Several possibilities can explain this feature, especially considering that the mechanisms for the expression and modulation of thrombomodulin in vivo, a cofactor necessary for protein C activation, is poorly understood as are the other mechanisms for the clearance of activated protein C. A theoretical disappearance half-life of about 76 minutes has been suggested for activated protein C in man and thus it is not surprising that in presence of normal synthetic liver function, the organism is able to compensate the decreased turnover of this inhibitor (Strickland and Kessler, 1987). Moreover, both immunological and functional assays measure also activated protein C.

Step 5: Low plasminogen level, low α-2-antiplasmin level, shortened survival of α-2-antiplasmin and increased levels of plasmin-α-2-antiplasmin complexes have been consistently found in AL with DIC (Kahlè et al., 1985; Bratt et al., 1985; Avvisati et al., 1988). All these changes can be predicted as a consequence of secondary activation of fibrinolysis. That fibrinolysis is not a primitive event but is secondary to activation of clotting system is well documented by the recent availability of methods employing monoclonal antibodies, which can discrimined between fibrinogen and fibrin degradation products. We are refering to the measurement of cross-linked fragments D (D-dimer). D-dimer is a marker of digestion of cross-linked fibrin and is not produced by degradation of fibrinogen and can be directly assayed in patient's plasma. We have invariably found a marked increased D-dimer level in all the cases in which the usual FDP test in serum was positive (>10 µg/ml). In any case, a lytic state has not been found in acute leukemia (Guarini et al. 1987b).

Thrombocytopenia is not usually considered among the laboratory manifestations of DIC in AL, since a low count might depend on marrow failure, rather than peripheral consumption due to trapping into the fibrin network of microthrombi. Nevertheless, we thought interesting to compare platelet count found at diagnosis in unselected cases of APL in comparison with AML and ALL. As can be shown in table 5, platelet count is greatly reduced in APL, as is fibrinogen level.

Table 5. Mean fibrinogen and platelet count at diagnosis in patients with acute leukemia of different types

	Fibrinogen (mg/dL)	Platelet ($10/\mu L$)
AML (91 cases)	301 (104)	79 (78)
ALL (49 cases)	316 (113)	78 (79)
APL (62 cases)	144 (78)**	35 (35) **

** $P < 0.01$ APL vs. AML and ALL

Reduced platelet count in APL, apart from its pathophysiological significance, seems also important from the clinical point of view since the lower platelet count, associated to reduced fibrinogen, might per se contribute to the severe hemorrhages observed in APL.

In summary, the complex pattern of clotting abnormalities observed in AL is in keeping with a pathogenetic mechanism which implies thrombin generation. None of the suggested alternative mechanisms (primary fibrinolysis or proteolysis) explain all the observed abnormalities. However, the contribution of these mechanisms to "DIC" can not be completely ruled out in the individual patient.

PROGNOSIS AND THERAPY

The occurrence of DIC in AL is probably a major risk factor for severe hemorrhagic manifestations both in AML and ALL. However, apart from the promyelocytic type, the prognostic significance of clotting abnormalities in AL is poorly understood, due to the relative rarity of DIC.

On the contrary, in APL, in which DIC is almost invariably present, an increased risk of hemorrhagic deaths, before or during induction therapy, has been well documented and has been recognized since the early reports (Rosenthal, 1963). The prevalence of hemorrhagic deaths in APL occurring during inductive therapy in patients treated after 1973 with anthracycline-containing regimens are presented in table 6:

Table 6. Hemorrhagic deaths in APL during inductive therapy
(Anthracycline-containing regimens only)

	HEPARIN		NO HEPARIN	
	n	deaths	n	deaths
Drapkin, 1978	9	2	15	9
Ruggero, 1977	0	-	13	4
Daly, 1980	10	1	5	1
Collins, 1978	7	1	0	-
Bernard, 1973	9	4	35	9
Cordonnier, 1985	57	6	0	-
Cunningham, 1984	50	6	3	0
Kantarjian, 1986	31	6	28	9
Goldberg, 1987	2	0	25	4
Petti, 1987	12	1	48	4
Sanz, 1988	34	3	0	-
Hoyle, 1988	35	3	80	26
TOTAL	256	33 (13%)	252	66 (26%)*

* $P < 0.1$

Between 13 to 26% of cases, depending on whether heparin was used or not during induction, died from hemorrhage almost exclusively from cerebral origin. With the present remission rate between 60 to 80% (Champlin & Gale, 1987), hemorrhagic deaths thus represent a major cause of treatment failure. In reviewing our cases treated with an antracycline-containing regimen, we found 6 hemorrhagic-related deaths among 42 patients, despite routine administration of platelet concentrates and heparin in most cases.

Whereas it is well known that APL is complicated by an increased frequency of early fatal hemorrhages, it is not well established which hemostatic parameter could represent a reliable prognostic index for the risk of fatal hemorrhage. Table 7 summarizes laboratory parameters found to represent specific risk factors of hemorrhage in APL:

Table 7. Risk factors of hemorrhage in APL

- Low fibrinogen (Bernard et al, 1973, Hoyle et al, 1988)

- Thrombocytopenia (Kantarjian et al, 1986)

- Prolonged prothrombin time (Hoyle et al., 1988)

- High blast cell count, anemia, old age (Kantarjian et al, 1986)

- Decreased α-2-antiplasmin (Avvisati et al, 1988)

- Defective fibrin cross-linking (Rodeghiero et al, 1984a)

No general agreement has been reached on a single hemostatic parameter as a reliable indicator of hemorrhagic risk. A more favourable outcome has been associated with an initial plasma fibrinogen concentration greater than 100 mg% and low blast count (Bernard et al., 1973). The worse prognostic significance of low fibrinogen (150 mg% taken as discriminant value) was confirmed using multivariate analysis of pretreatment patient characteristics by Kantarjian et al (1986) in a series of 60 patients with APL, whereas the level of FDP had not a significant prognostic value. Other bad prognostic indexes were thrombocytopenia (< 30,000/µl), absolute blast count (higher than 1,000/µl), old age (> 50), hemoglobin (< 11 gr%) and presence of hemorrhagic symptoms. However, recently Sanz et al (1988) in a study of 34 cases of APL were not able to demonstrate increased risk of fatal hemorrhages in patients with overt DIC, a finding in accordance with the experience of Marty et al (1984) in their large serie of 119 patients with APL. In addition, other peculiar abnormalities not routinely investigated, such as defective fibrin cross-linking or decreased α-2-antiplasmin, may significantly contribute (Rodeghiero et al., 1984a; Avvisati et al., 1988).

THERAPY

The therapy of DIC in AL aims at reducing the risk of major hemorrhagic symptoms. Since the recognition of DIC in AL in early '60, heparin therapy was used in accordance with the current accepted therapeutic management of DIC. The ability of heparin to partially correct hypofibrinogenemia and thrombocytopenia in APL has been demonstrated since the early studies in the '60 (Baker at al., 1964). DIC in APL often worsens after starting of chemotherapy and heparin has been shown to be able to avoid rapid defibrination (Gralnick et al., 1972). This is in keeping with our experience: infusion at about 300 U/kg/day was able to avoid fibrinogen drop after chemotherapy (table 8).

Table 8. Fibrinogen level at diagnosis and 48 hr after starting chemotherapy in APL treated or not with heparin

	At diagnosis	During chemotherapy
WITH HEPARIN (n= 17)	143.5 (78.3)	152.9 (91.1)
SUPPORTIVE THERAPY ONLY (n= 33)	140.9 (81.9)	112.1 (77.4)*

P < 0.05 versus cases treated with heparin

Despite heparin is no longer advised as routine treatment of DIC, its use in APL has persisted and is still suggested as the first choice treatment in major textbooks (Wintrobe et al., 1981; Williams et al., 1983), even if no prospective randomized studies are available to demonstrate its beneficial effect. The cumulative results of historical series of patients with APL treated with antracycline-containing regimens including or not heparin during induction, are reported in table 9.

Table 9. Effect of heparin on the complete remission (CR) rate in APL
(Anthracycline-containing regimens only)

	HEPARIN		NO HEPARIN	
	n	CR	n	CR
Drapkin, 1978	9	7	8	2
Ruggero, 1977	0	-	13	4
Daly, 1980	10	8	5	3
Collins, 1978	7	5	0	-
Bernard, 1973	9	3	35	16
Cordonnier, 1985	57	30	0	-
Cunningham, 1984	54	41	3	2
Kantarjian, 1986	31	18	28	14
Goldberg, 1987	2	1	25	19
Petti, 1987	12	6	48	38
Sanz, 1988	34	23	0	-
Hoyle, 1988	35	30	80	39
TOTAL	260	172 (66%)	245	140 (57%)

A favourable trend, although not statistically significant, is evident for heparin treated patients in terms of both complete remission rate and hemorrhagic deaths (table 9).

Perplexities in the use of heparin in the treatment of hemorrhagic complications of APL are due to remain until a prospective randomized study will adress the problem. Some authors think that excessive fibrinolysis (whether primitive or not) is a definite cause of bleeding in these patients. Reduced α-2-antiplasmin level was suggested as a reliable indicator of hemorrhagic risk and administration of antifibrinolytic agents was shown to be able to control bleeding symptoms and to restore severely reduced level of this plasmin inhibitor (Schwartz et al., 1986; Avvisati et al., 1988). However, cases of APL treated with antibrinolytic agents remains sporadic and no definite conclusion can be drawn (Keane et al., 1976; Talarico and Weintraub, 1977; Chan et al., 1984). In any case, the well documented evidence of thrombotic complication occurring after the administration of these agents (Schwartz et al., 1986) should make mandatory the concomitant administration of heparin.

At present, in the management of DIC in AL, especially in APL, substitutive therapy with platelet and plasma transfusion immediately after diagnosis remains of fundamental importance. Platelet count should be maintained above 50,000/µl and fibrinogen above 100 mg% (Bernard et al., 1973; Kantarjian et al., 1986).

CONCLUSIONS AND DIRECTIONS FOR FUTURE INVESTIGATIONS

A large body of evidence indicates that thrombin is generated in blood during DIC in AL. On the basis of this hypothesis a clear understanding of the clotting abnormalities usually found in AL can be offered and high procoagulant potential has been generally found in leukemic cells. Further characterization of procoagulant and fibrinolytic activities of blast cells is required in order to have a better understanding of the trigger mechanism of DIC. With the present available methodology the diagnosis of DIC remains largely operational and, thus, the contribution to the observed clotting abnormalities of primary fibrinolysis or proteolysis can not be excluded in the individual patient. Moreover, since the upmost part of leukemic mass is endowed outside the vascular compartment, the possibility of extravascular thrombin generation should not be overlooked. In this regard we need a more complete knowledge about biological mechanisms related to blood-marrow barrier. No single hemostatic parameter is reliable prognostic indicator of early death. Substitutive therapy with plasma, cryoprecipitate and platelet transfusions remains fundamental and should be instituted as soon as possible. The effectiveness of heparin remains to be clearly demonstrated by future controlled prospective studies even if a favourable trend has been noted in several clinical studies.

REFERENCES

Al-Mondhiry, H., Lawlor, D., Sadula, D. (1975a): Fibrinogen survival and fibrinolysis in acute leukemia. Cancer 35, 432-435.
Al-Mondhiry, H. (1975b): Disseminated intravascular coagulation. Experience in a major cancer center. Thrombos. Diathes. haemorrh. 34, 181-193.
Arlin, Z.A., Kempin, S., Mertelsmann, R., Gee, T., Higgins, C., Jhanwar, S., Chaganti, R.S.K., Clarkson, B. (1984): Primary therapy of acute promyelocytic leukemia: results of amsacrine- and daunorubicin-based therapy. Blood 63, 211-212.
Avvisati, G., ten Cate, J.W., Lamping, R., Petti, M.C., Mandelli, F. (1988): Acquired α-2-antiplasmin deficiency in acute promyelocytic leukemia. Br. J. Haematol., in press.
Baker, W., Bang, N.U., Nachman, R.L., Raafat, R., Horowitz, H.I. (1964): Hypofibrinogenemic hemorrhage in acute myelogenous leukemia treated with heparin. Ann. Intern. Med. 61, 116-123.
Barbui, T., Battista, R., Dini, E. (1976): Fibrinogen survival with seleniomethionine in acute myeloblastic leukemia during polychemotherapy. Haematologica 61; 73-80.
Bastard, C., Vannier, J.P., Bizet, M., Leonormand, B., Tron, P. (1985): Translocation (4;11;17) in a case of acute lymphoblastic leukemia. Cancer Gen. Cytogen. 17, 81-82.
Bauer, K.A., Rosenberg, R. (1984): Thrombin generation in acute promyelocytic leukemia. Blood 64, 791-796.
Bennet, M., Parker, A.C., Ludlam, C.A. (1976a): Platelet and fibrinogen survival in acute promyelocytic leukaemia. Br. Med. J. ii, 565.
Bennet, J.M., Catovsky, D., Daniel, M.T., Flandrin, G., Galton, D.A.G.,

Gralnick, H.R., Sultan, C. (1976b): Proposal for the classification of the acute leukaemias. Br. J. Haematol. 33, 451-458.

Bernard, J., Mathe, G., Boulay, J., Ceoara, B., Chome J. (1959): Le leucemie aigue a promyelocytes. Etude portant sur vingt observations. Schw. Med. Wochens. 89, 604-608.

Bernard, J., Weil, M., Boiron, M., Jacquillat, C., Flandrin, G., Gemon, M.F. (1973): Acute promyelocytic leukemia: results of treatment by daunorubicin. Blood 41, 489-496.

Brakman, P., Snyder, J., Enderson, E.S., Astrup, T. (1970): Blood coagulation and fibrinolysis in acute leukemia. Br. J. Haematol. 18, 135-145.

Bratt, G., Blomback, M., Paul, C., Schulman, S., Tornebohm, E., Lockner, D. (1985): Factors and inhibitors of blood coagulation and fibrinolysis in acute non-lymphoblastic leukaemia. Scand. J. Haematol. 34, 332-339.

Champion, L.A.A., Luddy, R.E., Schwartz, A.D. (1978): Disseminated intravascular coagulation in childhood acute lymphocytic leukemia with poor prognostic features. Cancer 41, 1642-1646.

Champlin, R., Gale, R.P. (1987): Acute myelogenous leukemia: Recent advances in therapy. Blood 69, 1551-1562.

Chan, T.K., Chan, G.T.C., Chan, Y. (1984): Hypofibrinogenemia due to increased fibrinolysis in two patients with acute promyelocytic leukemia. Aust. N. Zeal. J. Med. 14, 245-249.

Chorba, T.L., Orenstein, J.M., Ney, A.B., Schwartz, B.S., Alabaster, O., Cohen, P. Kessler, C.M., , Schulof, R.S. (1985): Phenotypic and ultrastructural characterization of a medullary thymocyte acute lymphoblastic leukemia with cellular procoagulant activity. Cancer 55, 675-681.

Collins, A.J., Bloomfield, C.D., Peterson, B.A., McKenna, R.W., Edson, J.R. (1978): Acute promyelocytic leukemia: management of the coagulopathy during daunorubicin-prednisone remission induction. Arch. Intern. Med. 138, 1677-1680.

Cordonnier, C., Vernant, J.P., Brun, B., Gouault-Heilmann, M., Kuentz, M., Bierling, P., Farcet, J.P., Rodet, M., Duedari, N., Imbert, M., Jouault, H., Mannoni, P., Reyes, F., Dreyfus, B., Rochant, H. (1985): Acute promyelocytic leukemia in 57 previously untreated patients. Cancer 55, 18-25.

Cunningham, I., Gee, T., Kempin, S., Clarkson, B. (1984): Acute promyelocytic leukemia (APL): ten years experience. Proc. Am. Soc. Clin. Oncol. 3, 203.

Daly, P.A., Schiffer, C.A., Wiernik, P.H. (1980): Acute promyelocytic leukemia: clinical management of 15 patients. Am. J. Hematol. 8, 347-359.

Daly, P., Brito-Babapulle, V., Lawlor, E., Blaney, C., Parreira, A., Catovsky, D. (1986): Variant translocation t(8;22) and abnormalities of chromosome 15(q22) and 17(q12-21) in a Burkitt's lymphoma/leukaemia with disseminated intravascular coagulation. Br. J. Haematol. 64, 561-569.

Dewald, B., Rindler-Ludwig, R., Bretz, U., Baggiolini, M. (1975): Subcellular localization and heterogeneity of neutral proteases in neutrophilic polymorphonuclear leukocytes. J. Exp. Med. 141, 709-723.

Didisheim, P., Trombold, J.S., Vandervoort, R.L.E., Sougin Mibashan, R. (1964): Acute promyelocytic leukemia with fibrinogen and factor V deficiencies. Blood 23, 717-728.

Donati, M.B., Gambacorti-Passerini, C., Casali, B., Falanga, A., Vannotti, P.,

Fossati, G., Semeraro, N., Gordon, S.G. (1986): Cancer procoagulant in human tumor cells: evidence from melanoma patients. Cancer Res. 46, 6471-6474.

Drapkin, R.L., Gee, T.S., Dowling, M.D., Arlin, Z., McKenzie, S., Kempin, S., Clarkson, B. (1978): Prophylactic heparin therapy in acute promyelocytic leukemia. Cancer 41, 2484-2490.

Dvorak, H.F., Senger, D.R., Dvorak, A.M. (1983): Fibrin as a component of the tumor stroma: origin and biological significance. Canc. Metast. Rev. 2, 41.

Egbring, R., Schmidt, W., Fuchs, G., Havemann, K. (1977): Demonstration of granulocytic proteases in plasma of patients with acute leukemia and septicemia with coagulation defects. Blood 49, 219-231.

Eiseman, G., Stefanini, M. (1954): Thromboplastic activity of leukemic white cells. Proc. Soc. Exp. Biol. Med. 86, 763.

Falanga, A., Gordon, S.G. (1985): Isolation and characterization of cancer procoagulant: a cysteine proteinase from malignant tissue. Biochemistry 24, 5558-5567.

Falanga, A., Alessio, M.G., Donati, M.B., Barbui, T. (1988): A new procoagulant in acute leukemia. Blood 71, 870-875.

French, A.J., Lilleyman, J.S. (1979): Bleeding tendency of T-cell lymphoblastic leukemia. Lancet ii, 469-470.

Goldberg, M.A., Ginsburg, D., Mayer, R.J., Stone, M.R., Maguire, M., Rosenthal, D.S., Antin, J.H. (1987): Is heparin administration necessary during induction chemotherapy for patients with acute promyelocytic leukemia ? Blood 69, 187-191.

Golomb, H.M., Rowley, J.D., Vardiman, J.W., Testa, J.R., Butler, A. (1980): "Microgranular" acute promyelocytic leukemia: a distinct clinical, ultrastructural and cytogenetic entity. Blood 55, 253-259.

Gordon, S.G., Cross, B.A. (1981): A factor X activating cysteine protease from malignant tissue. J. Clin. Invest. 67, 1655-1671.

Gordon, S.G., Hashiba, U., Poole, M.A., Cross, B.A., Falanga, A. (1985): A cysteine proteinase procoagulant from amnion-chorion. Blood 66, 1261-1265.

Gouault-Heilmann, M., Chardon, E., Sultan, C., Josso, F. (1975): The procoagulant factor of leukaemic cells: demonstration of immunologic cross-reactivity with human brain tissue factor. Br. J. Haematol. 30, 151-158.

Gralnick, H.R., Bagley, J., Abrell, E. (1972a): Heparin treatment for the hemorrhagic diathesis of acute promyelocytic leukemia. Am. J. Med. 52, 167-174.

Gralnick, H.R., Marchesi, S., Givelber, H. (1972): Intravascular coagulation in acute leukemia: clinical and subclinical abnormalities. Blood 40, 709-718.

Gralnick, H.R., Abrell, E. (1973): Studies of the procoagulant and fibrinolytic activity of promyelocytes in acute promyelocytic leukaemia. Br. J. Haematol. 24, 89-99.

Gralnick, H.R., Sultan, C. (1975): Acute promyelocytic leukaemia: haemorrhagic manifestations and morphologic criteria. Br. J. Haematol. 29, 373-376.

Griffin, J.H., Mosher, D.F., Zimmerman, T.S., Kleiss, A.J. (1982): Protein C, an antithromboti protein, is reduced in hospitalized patients with intravascular coagulation. Blood 60, 261-264.

Groopman, J., Ellman, L. (1979): Acute promyelocytic leukemia. Am. J.

Hematol. 7, 395-408.
Guarini, A., Baccarani, M., Corbelli, G., Gugliotta, L., Tura, S. (1980): Defibrination in adult acute lymphoblastic leukemia. Report of four cases. Nouv. Rev. Fr. Hematol. 22, 115-123.
Guarini, A., Gugliotta, L., Timoncini, C., Chetti, L., Catani, L., Russo, D., Tura, S. (1985): Procoagulant cellular activity and disseminated intravascular coagulation in acute non-lymphoid leukaemia. Scand. J. Haematol. 34, 152-156.
Guarini, A., Gugliotta, L., Valvassori, L., Bagnara, G.P., Timoncini, C., Motta, M.R., Chetti, L., Catani, L., Russo, D., Tura, S. (1986): Human myeloid precursor cells do not possess or produce procoagulant activity (PCA). Exp. Hematol. 14, 72-74.
Guarini, A., Gugliotta, L., Catani, L., Chetti, L., Macchi, S., Tura, S. (1987): Procoagulant cellular activity (PCA) in the classification of acute leukemia. Thromb. Res. 45, 545-552.
Guarini, A., Mussoni, L., Gugliotta, L., Chetti, L., Niewiarowski, T., Catani, L., Macchi, S., Donati, M.B., Tura, S. (1987b): Depressed fibrinolysis in patients with acute leukaemia. Br. J. Haematol. 66, 323-326.
Gugliotta, L., Viganò, S., D'Angelo, A., Guarini, A., Tura, S., Mannucci, P.M. (1984): High fibrinopeptide A (FPA) levels in acute non-lymphocytic leukemia are reduced by heparin administration. Thromb. Haemostas. 52, 301-304.
Hillestad, L.K. (1957): Acute promyelocytic leukemia. Acta Med. Scand. 49, 189-194.
Hoyle, C.F., Swirsky, D.M:, Freedman, L., Hayhoe, F.G.J. (1988): Beneficial effect of heparin in the management of patients with APL. Br. J. Haematol. 68, 283-289.
Kahle', L.H., Avvisati, G., Lamping, R.J., Moretti, T., Mandelli, F. (1985): Turnover of alpha-2-antiplasmin in patients with acute promyelocytic leukemia. Scand. J. Clin. Lab. Invest. 45, Suppl. 178, 75-80.
Kantarjian, H.M., Keating, M.J., Walters, R.S., Estey, E.H., McCredie, K.B., Smith, T., Dalton, W., Cork, A., Trujillo, J.M., Freireich, E.J. (1986): Acute promyelocytic leukemia. M.D. Anderson Hospital experience. Am. J. Med. 80, 789-797.
Keane, T.J., Gorman, A.M., O'Connell, L.G., Fennelly, J.J. (1976): Epsilon-aminocaproic acid in the management of acute promyelocytic leukemia. Acta Haematol. 56, 202-204.
Lyberg, T., Ivhed, I., Prydz, H., Nilsson, K. (1983): Thromboplastin as a marker of monocyte differentiation. Br. J. Haematol. 53, 327-335.
Marty, M., Ganem, G., Fischer, J., Flandrin, G., Berger, R., Schaison, G., Degos, L., Boiron, M. (1984): Leucemie aigue promyelocytaire: etude retrospective de 119 malades traitee par daunorubicine. Nouv. Rev. Fr. Hematol. 26, 371-378.
McKenna, R.W., Parkin, J., Bloomfield, C.D., Sundberg, R.D., Brunning, R.D. (1982): Acute promyelocytic leukaemia: a study of 39 cases with identification of a hyperbasophilic variant. Br. J. Haematol. 50, 201-214.
Merskey, C. (1973): Defibrination syndrome or...? Blood 41, 599-603.
Mimuro, J., Sakata, Y., Wakabayashi, K., Matsuda, M. (1987): Level of protein C determined by combined assays during disseminated intravascular coagulation and oral anticoagulation. Blood 69, 1704-1711.

Muller-Berghaus, G., Niepoth, M., Rabens-Alles, B., Rump, E., Murano, G. (1985): Normal antithrombin-III activity and concentration in experimental disseminated intravascular coagulation. Scand. J. clin. Lab. Invest. 45, Suppl. 178, 107-113.

Myers, T.J., Rickles, F.R., Barb, C., Cronlund, M. (1981): Fibrinopeptide A in acute leukemia: relationship of activation of blood coagulation to disease activity. Blood 57, 518-525.

Niemetz, J., Nossel, H.F. (1969): Activated coagulation factors: in-vivo and in-vitro studies. Br. J. Haematol. 16, 337-351.

Petti, M.C., Avvisati, G., Amadori, S., Baccarani, M., Guarini, A.R., Papa, G., Rosti, G.A., Tura, S., Mandelli, F. (1987): Acute promyelocytic leukemia: clinical aspects and results of treatment in 62 patients. Haematologica 72, 151-155.

Pogliani, E., Gambacorti-Passerini, C., Cofrancesco, E., Donati, M.B., Semeraro, N. (1986): Impaired generation of procoagulant activity in leukaemic monoblasts. Br. J. Haematol. 62, 197-199.

Quigley, H.J., (1967): Peripheral leukocyte thromboplastin in promyelocytic leukemia. Fed. Proc. 26, 648 (ab).

Rodeghiero, F., Barbui, T. (1977): Two dimensional immunoelectrophoresis of antithrombin III during disseminated intravascular coagulation in acute leukemia. Thromb. Res. 12, 191-196.

Rodeghiero, F., Barbui, T., Battista, R., Chisesi, T., Rigoni, G., Dini, E. (1980): Molecular subunits and transamidase activity of factor XIII during disseminated intravascular coagulation in acute leukemia. Thromb. Haemostas. 43, 6-9.

Rodeghiero, F., Morbin, M., Barbui, T. (1981): Subunit A of factor XIII regulates subunit B plasma concentration. Thromb. Haemostas. 46, 621-622.

Rodeghiero, F., Mannucci, P.M., Viganò, S., Barbui, T., Gugliotta, L., Cortellaro, M., Dini, E. (1984a): Liver dysfunction rather than intravascular coagulation as the main cause of low protein C and antithrombin III in acute leukemia. Blood 63, 965-969.

Rodeghiero, F., Barbui, T., Dal Belin Peruffo, A., Dini, E. (1984b): Defective fibrin cross-linking in acute leukemia. Thromb. Haemostas. 52, 343-346.

Rodeghiero, F., Castaman, G., Soffiati, G., Quaglio, R., Castronovo, S., Dini, E. (1988): Clinical significance of fibrinopeptide A in acute lymphocytic and non-lymphocytic leukemia. In press.

Rosenthal, R. (1963): Acute promyelocytic leukemia associated with hypofibrinogenemia. Blood 21, 495-508

Ruggero, D., Baccarani, M., Guarini, A. (1977): Acute promyelocytic leukemia: results of therapy and analysis of 13 cases. Acta Haematol. 58, 108-119.

Sakuragawa, N., Takahashi, K., Hoshiyama, M., Jimbo, C., Matsuoka, M., Onishy, J. (1976): Pathologic cells as procoagulant substance of disseminated intravascular coagulation syndrome in acute promyelocytic leukemia. Thromb. Res. 8, 263-273.

Sandler, R.M., Liebman, H.A., Patch, M.J., Teitelbaum, A., Levine, A.M., Feinstein, D.I. (1983): Antithrombin III and anti-activated factor X activity in patients with acute promyelocytic leukemia and disseminated intravascular coagulation. Cancer 51, 681-685

Sanz, M., Jargue, I., Martin, G., Lorenzo, I., Martinez, J., Rafecas, J., Pastor, E., Sayas, M.J., Sanz, G., Gomis, F: (1988): Acute promyelocytic leukemia. Therapy results and prognostic factors. Cancer 61, 7-13.

Schmidt, W., Egbring, R., Haveman, K. (1974): Effect of elastase-like and of chymotrypsin-like neutral proteases from human granulocytes on isolated clotting factors. Thromb. Res. 6, 315-321.

Schwartz, B.S., Williams, E.C., Conlan, M.G., Mosher, D.F. (1986): Epsilon-aminocaproic acid in the treatment of patients with acute promyelocytic leukemia and acquired -2-plasmin inhibitor deficiency. Ann. Intern. Med. 105, 873-877.

Sielgal. T., Seligsohn, U., Aghai, E., Modan, M. (1978): Clinical and laboratory aspects of disseminated intravascular coagulation (DIC): a study of 118 cases. Thromb. Haemostas. 39, 122-134.

Spero, J.A., Lewis, J.H., Hasiba, U. (1980): Disseminated intravascular coagulation. Findings in 346 patients. Thromb. Haemostas. 43, 28-33.

Strickland, D.K., Kessler, C.M. (1987): Biochemical and functional properties of protein C and protein S. Clin. Chim. Acta 170, 1-24.

Talarico, L., Weintraub, L.R. (1977): Leukocytic fibrinolysis in myelomonocytic leukemia. Cancer 39, 1618-1624.

Tanaka, K., Imamura, T. (1983): Incidence and clinicopathological significance of DIC in autopsy cases. In Disseminated Intravascular Coagulation, eds. T. Abe and M. Yamanaka, pp 79-86. Tokyo: University of Tokyo Press.

Vandewater, L., Tracy, P.B., Aronson, D., Mann, K.G., Dvorak, H.F. (1985): Tumor cell generation of thrombin via functional prothrombinase assembly. Cancer Res. 45, 5521-5525.

Verstrate, M., Vermylen, C., Vermylen, J., Vandenbroucke, S. (1965): Excessive consumption of blood coagulation components as cause of hemorrhagic diathesis. Am. J. Med. 38, 899-908.

Yoda, Y., Abe, T. (1981): Fibrinopeptide A (FPA) level and fibrinogen kinetics in patients with malignant disease. Thromb. Haemostas. 46, 706-709.

Wada, H., Nagano, T., Tomeoku, M., Kuto, M., Karitani, Y., Deguchi, K., Shirakawa, S. (1982): Coagulant and fibrinolytic activities in the leukemic cells lysates. Thromb. Res. 30, 315-322.

Williams, W.J., Beutler, E., Erslev, A.J., Lichtman, M.A. (eds) (1983): Hematology. New York: McGraw-Hill.

Wilson, E.L., Jacobs, P., Dowdle, E.B. (1983): The secretion of plasminogen activators by human myeloid leukemic cells in vitro. Blood 61, 568-574.

Wintrobe, M.M., Lee, G.R., Boggs, D.R., Birhell, T.C., Roerstor, J., Athons, J.W., Lukens, J.N. (eds) (1981): Clinical Hematology. Philadelphia: Lea and Febiger.

Activation of blood coagulation in the blast phase of chronic myelogenous leukemia

A. Sagripanti, F. Papineschi, E. Pinori*, M. Ferdeghini*

Servizio di Ematologia, Clinica Medica I e Servizio di Medicina Nucleare,
Università degli Studi di Pisa, Ospedale S. Chiara, via Roma, Pisa, Italy*

ABSTRACT

Fibrinopeptide A, a sensitive index of in vivo thrombin action on fibrinogen, beta--thromboglobulin and platelet factor 4, two platelet specific proteins considered to be indicators of the platelet release-reaction, have been measured in plasma by radioimmunoassays in 29 patients affected with chronic myelogenous leukemia (9 of them were in blast crisis, the others in chronic phase). Fibrinopeptide A (mean ± ± SD) was higher in blast phase (4.10 ± 3.26 ng/ml) than in chronic phase ($1.63 \pm \pm 0.63$ ng/ml; $p < 0.005$); also beta-thromboglobulin value was more elevated in blastic phase than in chronic phase, when corrected for platelet count (ratio: 59 ± 58 versus 19 ± 7; $p < 0.01$). Our data provide evidence of blood clotting activation during the blast phase of chronic myelogenous leukemia.

KEYWORDS

Blast phase of chronic myelogenous leukemia, hypercoagulability, fibrinopeptide A, beta-thromboglobulin, platelet factor 4.

INTRODUCTION

Thrombotic and haemorrhagic complications have been reported in chronic myelogenous leukemia (CML), expecially during the blast phase (Schafer, 1984). Aim of this study is to assess the degree of blood clotting activation in a series of patients affected with CML, in chronic phase or in blast crisis, by measuring plasmatic markers of in vivo haemostasis activation. fibrinopeptide A (FPA), a sensitive indicator of in vivo thrombin action on fibrinogen, has been determined in plasma by radioimmunoassay together with beta-thromboglobulin (BTG) and platelet factor 4 (PF4), two alpha granule platelet specific proteins known to be released in plasma during platelet stimulation.

MATERIAL AND METHODS

Patients

We have studied 29 patients affected with CML, 18 males and 11 females, aged 24 to 78 years. Twenty patients were in chronic phase; time from diagnosis of CML ranged from 1 month to 3 years; 5 of them had a prevous history of thrombotic disorders. Nine patients were in blast phase; diagnosis of blast phase was done by pertinent clinical and haematological data; all these subjects were examined in the early stage of blast crisis, before receiving any polichemotherapic regimen.

FPA, BTG and PF4 assays

Details concerning blood collection and subsequent manipulation of samples have been described elsewhere (Sagripanti, 1988); FPA, BTG and PF4 were measured in plasma by radioimmunoassays using commercial kits. Values were expressed as ng/ /ml (mean ± SD). BTG values were also corrected for platelet count according to Fabris (1984). Thirthy-two healthy subjects homogeneously matched with patients for age and sex were selected as controls; normal values are reported in table I.

Statistical analysis

All laboratory results were examined for significance using the Student's t-test and the Pearson's correlation test.

RESULTS

As it is reported in table I, plasma FPA levels were significantly more elevated in patients being in blast crisis (4.1 ± 3.3 ng/ml) than in patients examined during the chronic phase of CML (1.6 ± 0.6 ng/ml; $p < 0.01$); 8 out 9 subjects in blast crisis (89%) had FPA levels above the upper range of normals (mean ± 2 SD). Also the patients in the chronic phase of CML had raised plasma levels of FPA in comparison with normal controls ($p < 0.005$); in the chronic phase a positive correlation was found between FPA and plasma fibrinogen (Pearson's correlation coefficient 0.71; $p < 0.05$). A patient exhibited high plasma levels of FPA 3 and 2 months before the haematological diagnosis of blast crisis (5.04 and 5.55 ng/ml respectively); at the time of blast crisis FPA was 12.1 ng/ml. A subset of patients was available in whom FPA levels were determined both at the time of the haematological diagnosis of blast phase and thereafter as disease progressed: FPA levels increased significantly from 4.6 ± 3.9 ng/ml at diagnosis to 7.7 ± 2.5 ng/ml at preterminal stage ($p < 0.05$). Furthemore serial FPA determinations in a single patient, performed weekly, revealed a striking increase in FPA level (from 3.8 to 18.2 ng/ml) that was associated to clinical and instrumental evidence of splenic infarction; 7 days later FPA decreased to 4.1 ng/ml, paralleling clinical improvement.

Plasma levels of BTG were raised both in chronic phase (67 ± 47 ng/ml) and in blast crisis (101 ± 81 ng/ml) as compared to normal controls ($p < 0.001$), but there was no significant difference between chronic phase and blast phase. In chronic phase BTG was positively correlated to platelet count (r 0.76; $p < 0.001$), to PF4 (r 0.64; $p < 0.01$) and to serum lactic dehydrogenase (r 0.52; $p < 0.05$); on the other hand no relationship was found between BTG and FPA. BTG ratio, that is plasma BTG value corrected for platelet count, was significantly higher in blast phase than in chronic phase (table I); also the group of patients in chronic phase had increased BTG ratio values as compared to normal controls ($p < 0.05$).

Plasma levels of PF4 were elevated both in chronic phase and in blast crisis in comparison with controls ($p < 0.001$), as shown in table I; no statistical difference was found between the two groups of patients.

Table I. Plasma levels of fibrinopeptide A, beta-thromboglobulin and platelet factor 4, platelet count ($\times 10^9$/L) and BTG ratio values in 20 patients in chronic phase of CML, in 9 patients in blast crisis and in 32 healthy controls (values are expressed as mean ± SD).

	Chronic phase	Blast crisis	Controls	T-test (chronic vs blast phase)
FPA (ng/ml)	1.63±0.63	4.10±3.26	1.09±0.53	p < 0.01
BTG (ng/ml)	67±47	101±81	25.6±7.4	p NS
PF4 (ng/ml)	11.4±6.7	9.7±8.3	5.4±1.3	p NS
Platelet count	342±169	171±115	231±45	p < 0.01
BTG ratio	18.9±7.2	59±58	11.6±5.6	p < 0.01

DISCUSSION

Fibrinopeptide A is a 16-amino acid peptide cleaved from the A chain of fibrinogen by thrombin; since the plasma half-life for FPA is less than 4 min, plasma concentrations of the peptide reflect ongoing coagulation and so provide a kinetic measure of fibrinogen cleavage by thrombin (Nossel, 1976). An increased rate of fibrinogen turnover, elevated serum concentrations of fibrin degradation products and high plasma levels of FPA have been reported in the majority of patients affected with acute leukemia (Yoda,1981; Myers,1981). Furthemore, haematological remission was associated with a striking reduction in FPA levels, while relapse of acute leukemia was associated with abrupt increases in the generation of FPA in most individuals (Myers,1981). Procoagulant activities from malignant cells, such as tissue factor-like procoagulant, a factor VII-cofactor activating factor X and/or factor IX, as well as cancer procoagulant, a factor VII independent cysteine proteinase directly activating factor X, may account for blood hypercoagulability in acute leukemia (Gordon,1988). Scanty data on clotting activation are available concerning patients during the blast crisis of chronic myelogenous leukemia.

All the patients we have examined at the time of blast crisis diagnosis showed abnormally elevated FPA concentrations except one; serial FPA determinations revealed an upward trend in FPA level during the course of blastic phase, consistent with the evolution of haematological disease; moreover in a patient of our series increased FPA values preceded the onset of blast phase by a few months. Taken as a whole, these data suggest that plasma FPA could be evaluated as a marker of disease activity in the blast crisis of CML. The elevated FPA concentrations we have documented in blast crisis may be attributed to procoagulants from blast cells, according to the findings in acute leukemias (Myers,1981). The high FPA levels we have found also in the chronic phase of CML, although to a lesser extent, provide evidence of subclinical blood clotting activation.

With regard to platelet specific proteins, significantly raised BTG and PF4 plasma levels have been documented both in chronic and in blast phase; the pathogenetic mechanisms, however, seem to be different in the two groups of patients, as the different values of BTG ratio do suggest. High platelet counts appear to be responsible for BTG and PF4 increase in chronic phase; an accelerated platelet turnover may also play a role. On the other hand alpha granule leakage from defective or necrotic megakaryocytes as well as accelerated intravascular consumption of platelets may be responsible for BTG and PF4 increase in blast phase.

CONCLUSIONS

Our results provide evidence supporting the presence of enhanced blood coagulation during the blast crisis of chronic myelogenous leukemia and, to a lesser extent, in the course of chronic phase. The activation of the haemostatic system may play a role in the pathogenesis of thromboembolic complications; a decompensated intravascular coagulation with severe haemorrhages can also occur.

SUMMARY

To investigate haemostatic system activation in chronic myelogenous leukemia, we have measured in plasma by radioimmunoassays fibrinopeptide A, a specific marker of fibrinogen cleavage by thrombin, together with beta-thromboglobulin and platelet factor 4, two thrombocyte specific proteins released in plasma during platelet activation. Twenty-nine patients have been studied: 20 were in chronic phase, 9 in blast phase. Platelet count, plasma fibrinogen and serum lactic dehydrogenase have been also determined. In chronic phase patients FPA was enhanced as compared to normal controls, indicating blood hypercoagulability; the elevated BTG values were associated with high platelet counts. In blastic phase patients FPA levels and BTG ratio values (BTG concentrations corrected for platelet counts) were significantly increased not only versus controls, but also versus chronic phase patients: procoagulants from malignant cells may account for FPA increase; platelet and/or megakaryocyte defects may account for elevated BTG ratio. Our results indicate blood hypercoagulability in the blast crisis of CML and, to a lesser extent, during the chronic phase.

REFERENCES

Fabris,F., Randi,M.L., Casonato,A., Dal Bo Zanon,R., Bonvicini,P., Girolami,A. (1984): Clinical significance of beta-thromboglobulin in patients with high platelet count. Acta haemat. 71, 32-38.
Gordon,S.G., Falanga,A.(1988): Procoagulant factors in acute leukemia cells. Bergamo Spring Conferences on Hematology "Infections and haemorrhage in acute leukemia". Bergamo, June 13-14,1988, Abstract Book, p.11.
Myers,T.J., Rickles,F.R., Barb,C., Cronlund,M.(1981): Activation of blood coagulation in acute leukemia-fibrinopeptide A(FPA) generation. Blood 57, 518-525.
Nossel,H.L., Ti,M., Kaplan,K.L. et al.(1976):The generation of fibrinopeptide A in clinical blood samples.Evidence for thrombin activity. J.Clin.Invest.58, 1136-44.
Sagripanti,A., Cupisti,A., Ferdeghini,M., Pinori,E., Barsotti,G.(1988): Molecular markers of haemostasis activation in nephrotic syndrome. Nephron (in press).
Schafer,A.I.(1984): Bleeding and thrombosis in the myeloproliferative disorders. Blood 64, 1-12.
Yoda,Y., Abe,T.(1981): Fibrinopeptide A (FPA) level and fibrinogen kinetics in patients with malignant disease. Thromb.Haemostas. 46, 706-709.

Efficacy of human heat-treated antithrombin-III (At-III) in the management of disseminated intravascular coagulation (DIC) complicating acute leukemia

M. Bazzan, G. Tamponi, A. Fusaro, D. Marranca, C. Tarella

Dipartimento di Medicina ed Oncologia Sperimentale, Sezione di Ematologia, Università degli Studi di Torino, Torino, Italy

ABSTRACT

The efficacy of Antithrombin-III (At-III) in the management of disseminated intravascular coagulation (D.I.C.) was evaluated in 8 patients with acute leukemia. D.I.C. was the complication of an acute infectious process in 6 patients, while it was related to cellular lysis in the remaining two.
Human heat-treated At-III was administered together with low doses of heparin and, when required, with non-activated prothrombin complex and platelet transfusions.
The At-III containing regimen proved to be effective in 5 patients, whose haemocoagulative parameters were normalized within 48 hours of treatment, while no improvement was observed in 3 patients, who died for septic shock.
The results suggest that At-III may be an effective support for the recovery from D.I.C. complicating acute leukemia.

KEYWORDS

Antithrombin-III, management of D.I.C., acute leukemia.

INTRODUCTION

Disseminated intravascular coagulation (D.I.C.) is an important, life-threatening complication for patients with acute leukemia. D.I.C. more often ensues after massive release of procoagulant factors from leukemic cells lysed by chemotherapy (1). However, it can also occur during the aplastic phase, generally in association with an acute septic process (2).
Although several approaches have been attempted to improve the prognosis of D.I.C. complicating leukemia, an optimal regimen needs to be defined, so far. In particular, the use of heparin remains controversial due to its potential haemorragic risks. In addition, the efficacy of heparin is often impaired by the low

plasma levels of Antithrombin-III (At-III). In fact, management of D.I.C. with At-III has already been investigated, more extensively in animal models (3,4).

The recent availability of purified, heat-treated At-III (5) prompted us to evaluate the potential efficacy of this factor delivered in combination with heparin, in the treatment of leukemic patients with D.I.C. The use of At-III allowed to reduce heparin dosage, minimizing the haemorragic risks. Platelet tranfusions and non-activated prothrombin complex were administered as well, adjusting the delivery upon the haemocoagulative parameters. Eight patients were treated with the At-III containing regimen.

The results here presented suggest that At-III should be considered in view of a better management of leukemic patients with D.I.C..

MATERIALS AND METHODS

1) Patients

Eight adult patients with acute leukemia were studied (age:24-64). D.I.C. developed in 2 patients with acute non-lymphocytic leukemia (ANLL) at diagnosis (M5 and M3 subtype) during the first remission induction cycle (daunorubicin and ara-c). The remaining 6 patients (4 with ANLL and 2 with acute lymphocytic leukemia), had D.I.C. in association with an acute infection during the aplastic phase. Three out of these patients had leukemia at diagnosis, while the others were in their 2nd or 3rd relapse. The infectious process was sustained by gram negative sepsis in 2 patients and by fungal dissemination in one; in three patients the infectious agent could not be documented. Patients with aplasia received broad spectrum antibiotics (mezlocillin, vancomicin and amikacin) at the first febrile episode. Parenteral amphotericin B was added when fever lasted longer than 36-48 hours, in the absence of positive blood cultures.

2) Haemocoagulative tests

All patients were daily monitored with the following haemocoagulative tests: prothrombin time, thrombotest , aPTT, fibrinogen, FDP, At-III, d-dimer, platelet count.
Significative alterations of haemocoagulative tests were detected in all patients, when D.I.C. developed (see Table 1).

3) Treatment protocol.

As soon as D.I.C. was diagnosed the following substitutive regimen was instituted:
- heparin 100 U/kg i.v.b., b.i.d. for three days
- At-III 20 U/kg, i.v., b.i.d. for three days. Lyophylized heat-treated At-III was made available by Immuno (Pisa,Italy). No side effects were observed during At-III administration.
- prothrombin complex (Konyne,Cutter) 1000 U., b.i.d. when P.T. fell below 35%
- platelet transfusions, 8-10 U. p.d. when platelets were below 20.000/mmc.

TABLE 1 : HAEMOCOAGULATIVE PARAMETERS OF PATIENTS WITH D.I.C. BEFORE AND AFTER AT-III THERAPY.

PARAMETERS	VALUES(1)	
	before treatment(2)	after treatment(3)
PT (%)(4)	22-55	60-100
aPTT (sec)	40-55	35-45
fibrinogen (mg/dl)	85-150	120-240
At-III (%)(4)	35-65	75-130
FDP (ugr/ml)	25-180	0-25
d-dimer (ugr/ml)	750-1200	350-750

(1) results are expressed as range of values observed in the patients under study
(2) values refer to all patients studied
(3) values observed within 48 hours of therapy in the five patients who survived
(4) values express percent of standard control

RESULTS AND CONCLUSIONS

In three patients with chemotherapy induced aplasia no improvement of the acute coagulopathy was observed with our anti-D.I.C. protocol. In fact, although antibiotic treatment was promptly instituted, they remained febrile and died within 24-96 hours for septic shock and acute respiratory failure.
In the other 5 patients a rapid improvement of haemocoagulative parameters was observed no longer than 48 hours after institution of anti-D.I.C. treatment (see Table 1). Consequently haemorragic symptoms disappeared and all 5 patients recovered from the acute syndrome.
Interestingly, our At-III containing regimen proved to be effective not only in patients with sepsis related D.I.C., but also in both patients with ANLL whose D.I.C. resulted from massive leukemic lysis. In addition, no acute haemorragic or thrombotic complications could be observed following the

concomitant administration of At-III, low dose heparin and non-activated prothrombin complex.

The use of lyophylized heat-treated At-III allows to avoid excessive plasma transfusions, in patients receiving high total fluid input. Moreover, the exact amount of At-III administered can be recorded. Finally, heat-treated At-III has been proved to be safe for virus transmission (5).

Our results, given these observations, support the emerging role of At-III in the management of thrombotic and haemorragic manifestations of D.I.C. (6).

REFERENCES :

1) Niiya K.,Mitani M.,Taguchi H.,Hirose S.,Yamato K.,Fujishita M.,Yoshimoto S.,Kubonishi I.,Miyoshy I.(1984): Hypercoagulable state induced by combination chemotherapy in patients with acute leukemia. Thromb.Haemost.51:409.

2) Dale D.C.,Petersdorf R.G.(1987): Septic shock.in Harrison's Principles of Internal Medicine,Mc Graw Hill Book Co.,New York,pg 474-478.

3) Muller-Berghaus G.,Niepoth M.,Rabens-Alles B.,Rump E.,Murano G. (1983): Antithrombin III concentration and antithrombin III substitution in experimental disseminated intravascular coagulation. Thromb.Haemost.50:323.

4) Triantaphyllopulos D.C.(1984): Effects of human Antithrombin III on martality and blood coagulation induced in rabbits by endotoxin. Thromb.Haemost.51:232-236.

5) Tabor E.,Murano G.,Snoy P.,Gerety R.J.(1981): Inactivation of hepatitis B virus by heat in Antithrombin III stabilized with citrate.Thromb.Res.22:233-238

6) Blauhut B.,Kramar H.,Vinazzer H.,Bergmann H.(1985): Substitution of Antithrombin III in shock and DIC: a randomized study. Thromb.Res.39:81-89

Infections and haemorrhage in acute leukaemia, T. Barbui, A. Falanga, B. Minetti, S. Gorini, G. Tognoni and M.D. Donati, eds. John Libbey Eurotext, Paris © 1989, pp. 73-76

Is heparin necessary in the treatment of acute progranulocytic leukemia ?

G.P. Canellos

Dana-Farber Cancer Institute, Boston, Massachusetts, U.S.A.

RESUME

Acute progranulocytic leukemia is unique amongst the leukemias in that the malignant progranulocytes contain procoagulant substances within the excessive number of granules that characterize that form of leukemia. Elaboration of these substances into the serum are associated with a picture of disseminated intravascular coagulation. Although the mechanism is now well known, the appropriate treatment is not clear. Prompt and aggressive therapy of the leukemic process results in exacerbation of the intravascular coagulation over a few days but is followed by rapid improvement. The use of heparin as part of the induction treatment is controversial and a critical review of the literature shows that treatment programs with heparin does not seem to offer a therapeutic survival advantage over those who do not use heparin. At the present time, the administration of heparin at low dose does not seem to be essential for the appropriate treatment of acute progranulocytic leukemia. If heparin is used, very low doses are probably inappropriate.

KEYWORDS

Heparin, Acute Progranulocytic Leukemia

Acute progranulocytic leukemia has been known as a distinct entity since 1957. It has unique features characterized by the presence of excessive granules in cells definable as progranulocytes and has been further subclassified according to the character of the granules into the microgranular or macrogranular variants. In addition, this disorder has a unique chromosomal abnormality characterized by a translocation of genetic chromosomal material between chromosomes #15 and #17 (t15:17). The exact role of this translocation in the pathogenesis of the disease is unknown. The original descriptions of the disorder also defined a high incidence of hemorrhagic complications, and it was early speculated that there was a measure of disseminated intravascular coagulation associated with the excessive proliferation of neoplastic progranulocytes (Gralnick and Sultan, 1975; Didisheim et al, 1964). The elaboration of procoagulant factors by the granules was postulated as the principal pathogenetic mechanism (Gralnick et al, 1972). The fact that exacerbation of the coagulopathy could occur with the initiation of therapy presumably by the destruction of a large number of malignant cells further suggested the above mechanisms. The early descriptions also reported a high incidence of hemorrhagic deaths, especially intracerebral hemorrhage. Although it was speculated that disseminated intravascular coagulation was the key mechanism, it wasn't until the last 15 years that careful coagulation studies demonstrated that there was a consumption of coagulant protein as well as an increased production of fibrinogen degradation products. Detailed studies using sensitive radio-immunoassays have demonstrated evidence of increased thrombin generation. This is characterized by increases in the measurable quantities of prothrombin scission protein, F1 and 2, as well as increases in the presence of complexes of thrombin and its inhibitor antithrombin (T-AT) (Bauer and Rosenberg, 1984). Early investigations of the drug, daunorubicin, demonstrated a high order of sensitivity of acute progranulocytic leukemia with a 50% complete remission rate. This agent has remained the mainstay of therapy in acute progranulocytic leukemia and its combination with cytosine arabinoside have been widely used in most trials (Bernard et al, 1973). Improvement in complete remission rate and disease-free survival cannot be attributed only to the successful chemotherapy. The availability of appropriate blood products, including fresh frozen plasma and platelet concentrates, has also made its contribution to the improved results.

The role of heparin has been controversial, and since the presumed association of disseminated intravascular coagulation with this disease, there has been a fashion for using low-dose heparin in some series. In fact, many series would suggest that it is standard practice to include heparin. Because of the high propensity for leukemic patients to bleed, there has also been a natural hesitation about the use of heparin in newly-diagnosed patients with acute progranulocytic leukemia. In the total absence of randomized clinical trials, individual institutional series have/have not employed heparin as part of initial management. Therefore, there is no scientific body of evidence that defends the use of heparin as part of the treatment of the disease. It would appear that the rapid elimination of leukemic progranulocytes is paramount to the arresting of the procoagulant process. In fact, detailed studies of fibrinogen degradation products have shown an early enhancement of disseminated intravascular coagulation within two days of therapy followed by rapid correction of the coagulation abnormalities (Bauer et al, 1984). There is clearly no significant difference in complete remission rate or hemorrhagic deaths amongst the series. Thirty-four patients with acute progranulocytic leukemia have been treated at the Dana-Farber Cancer Institute and the Brigham and Women's Hospital since 1975. Despite the fact that 29/34 (85%) had laboratory evidence of coagulation abnormality, all but six cases received no heparin as part of the induction therapy. All patients were treated with an anthracycline antibiotic and cytosine arabinoside. The complete remission rate was 74% (Goldberg et al, 1987; Stone et al, 1988). A compilation of the experience with the use with/without heparin in remission induction in progranulocytic leukemia is shown on Table 1.

It would appear that a critical mass of leukemic progranulocytes is probably essential for the genesis of the pattern of diffuse intravascular coagulation. A phenomenon fairly unique to the therapy of acute leukemia has been observed in the management of acute progranulocytic leukemia. As opposed to most forms of acute leukemia where aplasia must be achieved to achieve a remission, this does not seem to be the case in acute progranulocytic leukemia. This study was made by observation of serial bone marrow specimens following the induction of therapy. Patients who by Day 15 still have residual abnormal progranulocytes as well as adequate cellularity might be considered having achieved an inadequate anti-leukemic response and could be, therefore, retreated. The experience at the Dana-Farber Cancer Institute and the Brigham and Women's Hospital suggested that these findings in the bone marrow do not necessarily indicate a failure of anti-leukemic therapy. The significance of these residual progranulocytes is unclear. The abnormal progranulocytes persisted in 17/25 complete remission patients even after a second induction course of chemotherapy.

Their persistence, however, did not appear to influence the coagulopathy since there was a diminished mass of these cells. They may represent end-stage differentiated cells of low turnover.

The isue of heparin administration as part of induction therapy for APL has not been resolved by any current trial. The data from the Dana-Farber Cancer Institute and Brigham and Women's Hospital as well as those other series were heparin was not used, would suggest that it is not essential or even life-saving. The determinants for risk of serious or fatal hemorrhage are many, but many include age, vascular fragility, platelet count, total mass of malignant progranulocytes, and duration prior to diagnosis. It is clear that the pattern of referral as well as socio-demographic factors which contribute to delay in diagnosis can influence the incidence of hemorrhagic death.

Table 1. Acute Progranulocytic Leukemia: Incidence of Complete Remission (CR) and Hemorrhagic Deaths (HD) with or without Heparin Administration*

	With Heparin			Without Heparin		
	No.	CR	HD	No.	CR	HD
Drapkin (1978)	9	7	0	8	2	5
Ruggero (1977)	0	-	-	13	7	4
Daly (1980)	10	8	1	5	3	1
Collins (1978)	7	5	1	0	-	-
Bernard (1973)	9	3	4	35	16	9
Cordonnier (1985)	57	30	15	0	-	-
Cunningham (1984)	54	41	7	3	2	1
Kantarjian (1986)	31	18	6	28	14	9
Goldberg (1987)	2	1	0	25	19	4
Sanz (1988)	34	23	3	0	-	-
TOTALS	213	136 (64%)	37 (17%)	117	63 (54%)	33 (28%)

* adapted from data in Goldberg et al, Blood 1987; 69, 187.

REFERENCES

Bauer, K.A. and Rosenberg, R.D. (1984): Thrombin generation in acute promyelocytic leukemia. Blood 64, 791-796.

Bernard, J., Weil, M., Boiron, M. et al (1973): Acute promyelocytic leukemia: Results of treatment by daunorubicin. Blood 41, 489-496.

Collins, A.J., Bloomfield, C.D., Peterson, B.A. et al (1978): Acute promyelocytic leukemia. Management of the coagulopathy during daunorubicin-prednisone remission induction. Arch. Intern. Med. 138, 1677-1680.

Cordonnier, C., Vernant, J.P., Brun, B. et al (1985): Acute promyelocytic leukemia in 57 previously untreated patients. Cancer 55, 18-25.

Cunningham, I., Gee, T., Kempin, S., and Clarkson, B. (1984): Acute promyelocytic leukemia (APL): Ten years experience. Proc. Am. Soc. Clin. Oncol. 3, 203.

Daly, P.A., Schiffer, C.A., Wiernik, P.H. (1980): Acute promyelocytic leukemia: Clinical management of 15 patients. Am. J. Hematol. 8, 347.

Didisheim, P., Trombold, J.S., Vandervoort, R.L.E., and Mibashan, R.S. (1964): Acute promyelocytic leukemia with fibrinogen and factor V deficiencies. Blood 23, 717-728.

Drapkin, R.L., Gee, T.S., Dowling, M.D., et al (1978): Prophylactic heparin therapy in acute promyelocytic leukemia. Cancer 41, 2484-2490.

Goldberg, M.A., Ginsburg, D., Mayer, R.J., et al (1987): Is heparin administration necessary during induction chemotherapy for patients with acute promyelocytic leukemia? Blood 69, 187-191.

Gralnick, H.R., Marchesi, S., and Givelber, H. (1972): Intravascular coagulation in acute leukemia: Clinical and subclinical abnormalities. Blood 40, 709-718.

Gralnick, H.R. and Sultan, C. (1975): Acute promyelocytic leukaemia: Haemorrhagic manifestation and morphologic criteria. Br. J. Haematol. 29, 373-376.

Kantarjian, H.M., Keating, M.J., Walters, R.S., et al (1987): Role of maintenance chemotherapy in acute promyelocytic leukemia. Cancer 59, 1258-1263.

Ruggero, D., Baccarani, M., Guarini, A., et al (1977): Acute promyelocytic leukemia: Results of therapy and analysis of 13 cases. Acta Hematol 58, 108.

Sanz, M.A., Jarque, I., Martin G., et al (1988): Acute promyelocytic leukemia. Cancer 61, 7-13.

Stone, R.M., Maguire, M., Goldberg, M.A., et al (1988): Complete remission in acute promyelocytic leukemia despite persistence of abnormal bone marrow promyelocytes during induction chemotherapy: Experience in 34 patient. Blood 71, 690-696.

Tranexamic acid versus placebo in treating the coagulopathy of acute promyelocytic leukemia

G. Avvisati, J.W. ten Cate[1], H.R. Büller[1], M.T. Petrucci, A. Spadea, F. Mandelli

Section of Hematology, Department of Human Biopathology, University «La Sapienza», Rome, Italy
[1] Center of Hemostasis Thrombosis and Atherosclerosis, Academic Medical Center, University of Amsterdam, The Netherlands

ABSTRACT

Between October 1985 and December 1987, 12 consecutive patients with acute promyelocytic leukemia were randomized to receive or not tranexamic acid in a double blind fashion and following an informed consent procedure. Objectives of the study were to verfy the effects of tranexamic acid on the incidence of hemorrhages and on the number of packet red cells transfused (PRC) as a measure of blood loss.
The number of hemorrhages and of PRC was significantly reduced in the tranexamic acid group. Therefore our data support the hypothesis that primary fibrinolysis is at least partially responsible for the bleeding tencency observed in acute promyelocytic leukemia and that tranexamic acid significantly reduces the hemorrhagic tendency observed in these patients.

KEY WORDS

Acute promyelocytic leukemia, coagulopathy, tranexamic acid

INTRODUCTION

Acute promyelocytic leukemia (APL) is a rare subtype of acute non lymphocytic leukemia with typical morphologic, cytogenetic, clinical and prognostic features. Since its first description it was associated with a severe coagulopathy presents in over 80%-90% of patients and responsible of the high mortality rate from massive brain hemorrhages observed during the first period following the diagnosis (Cordonnier et al, 1985; Kantarjian et al, 1986; Sanz et al, 1988).
The mechanism responsible of this coagulopathy has been attributed throughout the years to fibrinolysis, proteolysis or to an extrinsic activation of blood coagulation leading to disseminated intravascular coagulation (DIC). It is presumed that the release of activators of the fibrinolytic system and/or of proteases

and/or of thromboplastic material from the leukemic cells is responsible for the activation of the various system (Avvisati et al; 1987). However it has been generally accepted that the coagulopathy is mainly a consequence of DIC triggered by procoagulant substances released from the granules of the leukemic promyelocytes. Therefore, despite the absence of prospective randomized clinical trials showing a favourable effect of heparin on clinical outcome, heparin treatment is widely accepted as a corner stone in the treatment of the bleeding tendency observed in APL patients. Our data collected in recent years in 21 consecutive APL patients demonstrated that a severe alpha-2-antiplasmin deficiency is present in all APL patients as the major defect, while the antithrombin III as well as the protein C levels remained within the normal ranges (Avvisati et al; 1988) This reduction is secondary to an increased turnover of the major fibrinolytic inhibitor (Kahlé et al; 1985). Therefore we hypothesized that the alpha-2-antiplasmin deficiency together with thrombocytopenia is responsible of the severe bleeding tendency observed in APL which could be correctly treated by an antifibrinolytic agent as clearly showed in the congenital alpha-2-antiplasmin deficiency (Aoki et al,1980; Kluft et al, 1982). To clinical support this hypothesis we undertook a clinical trial in order to demonstrate in a double blind randomized fashion, the efficacy and safety of tranexamic acid in treating the bleeding diathesis of APL.

SUBJECTS AND METHODS

Between October 1985 and december 1987, 12 consecutive APL patients observed at the Institute of hematology of the University "La Sapienza" of Rome, were randomized to receive either tranexamic acid or placebo in a double blind fashion following an informed consent procedure. Tranexamic acid (6 g/daily) or placebo, were administered as continuous infusion for 6 days. An objective quantitation of hemorrhages as well as of the number of packed red cell (PRC) and platelet concentrate (PLT) transfusions was performed by a single investigator during a follow-up period of 7 days.

RESULTS

The number of PRC and PLT transfused was reduced in the tranexamic acid group. In particular 373 PLT were transfused in the tranexamic acid group versus 507 transfused in the control group. However this difference was not statistically significant. On the contrary, the reduction in the number of PRC transfused observed in the treated group was statistically significant (24 vs 39 PRC transfused in the treated and control group respectively; $P < 0.05$).
Significant was also the reduction in hemorrhages observed in the tranexamic acid group as compared to the placebo group (13 vs 40; $P < 0.05$).

CONCLUSIONS

This study demonstrates an important reduction in the bleeding diathesis and PRC requirement in APL patients treated with tranexamic acid. Therefore our data support the hypothesis that primary fibrinolysis is at least partially responsible for the bleeding tendency observed in APL and that treatment with tranexamic acid significantly reduces the hemorrhagic tendency in these patients.

REFERENCES

Aoki N., Sakata Y., Matsuda M., Tateno K. (1980): Fibrinolytic states in a patient with congenital deficiency of alpha-2-antiplasmin inhibitor. Blood 55, 483-488.

Avvisati G., ten Cate J.W., Mandelli F. (1987): The coagulopathy in acute promyelocytic leukemia: DIC? In Hemostasis and Cancer, ed L. Muzbeck pp 91-100. Boca Raton, Florida: CRC Press.

Avvisati G., ten Cate J.W., Sturk A., Lamping R., Petti M.C., Mandelli F. (1988): Acquired alpha-2-antiplasmin deficiency in acute promyelocytic leukaemia. Brit.J.Haematol 70, (in press).

Cordonnier C., Vernant J.P., Brun B. et al. (1985): Acute promyelocytic leukemia in 57 previously untreated patients. Cancer, 55; 18-25.

Kahlé L.H., Avvisati G., Lamping R.J., Moretti T., Mandelli F., ten Cate J.W. (1985): Turnover of alpha-2-antiplasmin in patients with acute promyelocytic leukemia. Scand.J.Clin.Lab.Invest. 45, (suppl. 148), 75-80.

Kantarjian H., Keating M.J., Walters R.S. et al (1986): Acute promyelocytic leukemia, M.D. Anderson hospital experience. Am.J.Med., 80, 789-797.

Kluft C., Vellenga E. Brommer E.J.P., Wijngaards G. (1982): A familial hemorrhagic diathesis in a Dutch family: an inherited deficiency of alpha-2-antiplasmin. Blood 59, 1169-1180.

Sanz M.A., Jarque I., Martin G., et al (1988): Acute promyelocytic leukemia. Therapy results and prognostic factors. Cancer, 61, 7-13.

Progressive induction for prevention of disseminated intravascular coagulation in acute promyelocytic leukemia : preliminary results

C. Cordonnier[1], F. Dreyfus, P. Casassus, V. Leblond, A. Pesce,
F. Teilletthibault, P. Colombat, X. Troussard, H. Dombret, M. Gouault,
H. Jouault, M. Kuentz, G. Karianakis, J.P. Vernant

[1] CHA, Promyelo Group, Hôpital Henri Mondor, 94000 Créteil, France

ABSTRACT

Thirty nine patients in first phase APL were treated with an original induction regimen consisting of daily increasing doses of chemotherapy to phase in progressively cytolysis of abnormal promyelocytes (CCNU, Daunomycin, Ara-C). All patients were given heparin (1 mg/kg/d) and platelet transfusions. When compared to an historical series of 57 patients treated with conventional therapy and the same management of disseminated intravascular coagulation (DIC), the complete remission rate raised from 53 % to 72 %, (n.s.) and the death rate during induction falled up from 47 % to 20 % (p<0.02). However, this was not associated with a different course of DIC, as far as fibrinogen and factor V levels were studied. Except for hyperleucocytic patients, gradual induction seems to be an interesting approach for the controle of DIC in APL. However, we have not the biological demonstration that the improvement of aplasia survival is due to a better controle of DIC. We are now beginning a randomized trial between conventional therapy and progressive induction.

KEY WORDS

Acute promyelocytic leukemia, progressive induction therapy.

INTRODUCTION

More than twenty years ago, acute promyelocytic leukemia (A.P.L.) has been isolated as a special form of acute myeloïd leukemia (AML), specially as regards to coagulation disorders and possible long term survival (Hillestad 1957, Bernard 1973). However, most of the teams dealing with AML have the same therapeutical approach for APL and other forms of AML, except for the use of heparin infusion, whose role has not been strongly demonstrated at the present time (Goldberg 1987, Hoyle 1988).

Because the intial prognosis of patients with APL seemed us being specially bad, we analyzed, in 1982, the charts of fifty seven patients in first phase APL who had been consecutively admitted and treated in our unit between 1972 and 1982 (Cordonnier 1985). This first study led us to conclude to :

- a complete remission (CR) rate of only 53 %
- a high (47 %) rate of death during induction, including early deaths (before

d5, 12 %) specially due to intracerebral hemorrhage, but also death during aplasia (after d5, 35 %).
- a relationship between the course of coagulation disorders during therapy and the occurrence of death during aplasia.

Renal and respiratory failure during induction were frequent in this series and, when an autopsy was obtained, were often associated with tissue damages suggestive for disseminated intravascular coagulation (DIC). However, we were unable to find any relationship between the occurrence of renal and respiratory failure and the initial severity of DIC. Therefore, we studied the evolution of DIC, specially of Fibrinogen and Factor V levels on d1, d3 and d5 during therapy and found that its worsening did significantly influence the occurrence of renal and respiratory failure. We hypothesized that the patients could suffer, during aplasia, from the late consequences of tissular DIC, specially on kidney and lung and, by analogy with Burkitt's lymphoma (Cohen 1980), could benefit from a more gradual induction to stagger the cytolysis, to make possible a better clearance of toxic products released by blast cells and by this way, to improve aplasia survival.

On the other hand, we had begun, in 1978, a new regimen for other AML, called "CHA", (Fig. 1) which gave encouraging results in terms of CR duration (Vernant 1987).

Figure 1 : INDUCTION THERAPY
           (mg/sq.m)

		D1	D2	D3	D4	D5	D6	D7	D8	D9	D10
CHAPROMYELO (APL)	Ara-C*	40	60	80	100	100	120	120	120	120	140
	Dauno	10	20	40	60	80	90				
	CCNU	40	40								
CHA (other AML)	Ara-C*	100	100	100	100	100	100	100	100	100	100
	Adria	35	35	35							
	CCNU	80									

*Continuous infusion

Therefore, the new protocole used for APL and started in 1983 took into account (1) the principle of progressive induction, (2) the general outline of CHA, with 10 days Ara-C. Thirty nine patients were treated with this regimen called 'CHA PROMYELO" between 1983 and 1988 and are analyzed in this report. This series is compared with (1) our first series of 57 APL patients treated between 1972-1982 with conventional therapy with 5 days Ara-C, (2) 121 patients with non M3-AML, treated with conventional CHA.

PATIENTS

Between 1/1983 and 2/1988, fifty one adults were consecutively identified as first phase APL according to the FAB classification (M3) in eight hematologic centers participating in the trial. Twelve of these patients were not enrolled in the study (early death due to intracerebral and/or intraalveolar hemorrhage : 2 ; cirrhosis : 1 ; severe chronic renal failure : 1 ; therapeutic mistakes according to the protocole : 3 (no heparin : 1, Doxomycin instead of Daunomycin : 2) ; age older than 65 and/or previous visceral failure leading to a less agressive regimen : 5). Thirty nine patients (Males : 16, Females : 23, mean age 39   13 years, extrems : 17-72) were finally included in this study and were given CHA-Promyelo. Five of them had previous malignancies treated with radiotherapy alone (n=2) or radio and chemotherapy (n=3).

The clinical characteristics of these 39 patients were comparable to those of our first series of APL (Table 1). The biological parameters at presentation were also comparable, except for the WBC count, which was higher in the first one (Table 2). By keeping the same criteria to define DIC than previously, the severity of DIC at presentation was identical before and after 1983 (Table 3).

TABLE 1 : CLINICAL CHARACTERISTICS AT PRESENTATION

	1972-1982	1983-1988
Cutaneous/mucous hemorrhages	77 %	77 %
Hemorrhagic fundus oculi	21 %	22 %
Fever > 38°C	53 %	54 %
Splenomegaly	5 %	13 %
Septic focus	21 %	23 %
Renal failure*	9 %	5 %
Respiratory failure**	7 %	0 %
Subarachnoid hemorrhage	2 %	0 %
	N = 57	N = 39

* defined by blood BUN > 0.8 g/l and urinary BUN < 15 g/l
** defined by a pAO_2 < 70 mmHg while breating room air

TABLE 2 : BIOLOGICAL CHARACTERISTICS AT PRESENTATION

Hemoglobin (g/dl)	9.5 ± 2.6	8.3 ± 1.7
Platelets ($\times 10^3/mm^3$)	39 ± 43	27 ± 18
WBC (")	20.3 ± 58.2	8 ± 20
WBC > 15,000/mm^3	13 (23 %)	3 (8 %)
Prothrombin time*	54 ± 20	60 ± 16
Factor V*	66 ± 29	79.5 ± 22
Fibrinogen (gm/dl)	299 ± 149	184 ± 092
	N = 57	N = 39

* % of normal

TABLE 3 - PARAMETERS AND SEVERITY OF DIC

INITIAL COAGULATION PARAMETERS		SEVERITY OF DIC AT PRESENTATION	
	CRITERIA	1972-1982 N=57	1983-1988 N=39
OVERT DIC	Fg < 0.2 gm/dl FactorV < 60 %	OVERT DIC 24 %	10.5 %
LATENT DIC	Fg < 0.2 gm/dl FactorV < 60 %	LATENT DIC 39 %	55 %
NO DIC	OTHER SITUATION	NO DIC 37 %	34.5 %

TREATMENT

1) Remission induction therapy.
CHA-Promyelo included Ara-C by continuous IV infusion, Daunomycin and CCNU (Fig.1). The total amount of drugs was the same as in conventional CHA given during the same time for the other forms of AML but with daily increasing doses of chemotherapy in CHA-Promyelo.

The protocole given to the first series of patients before 1982 associated 3 days of Daunomycin (100mg/sq.m/d) and 5 days of Ara-C (100 mg/sq.m/d) (Cordonnier 1985).

2) Supportive care
The patients were treated in private rooms with sterile food and gut sterilization. The management of DIC was exactly the same before and since 1983 and consisted of (1) platelet transfusions in order to maintain a platelet count above 60,000/mm^3 ; (2) systematic continuous heparin infusion at the initial dosage of 1 mg/kg/d, ultimately increased to 23 mg/kg if necessary according to the daily levels of fibrinogen and factor V. Heparin infusion was stopped between d10 and d15 after the beginning of chemotherapy.

3) Maintenance regimen.
Three weeks after achievement of CR with CHA-Promeylo, all the patients entered a three year maintenance regimen associating ; (1) every 3 months, periodic reinduction consisting of Daunomycin, CCNU and Ara-C, followed by 1 month rest ; (2) weekly combinations of 6-Thioguanine and Ara-C for 2 months.

RESULTS

1) Overall results with CHA Promyelo
Twenty eight (72 %) patients entered CR with one course of CHA Promyelo. Eleven patients relapsed between 5 to 24 months after achieving CR. Two patients died in CR (acute myocarditis : 1 ; post-hepatitic cirrhosis : 1). A plateau at 46 % seems to be obtained after the 24th month but the short follow up (48 months for the first patient included) led us to be cautious on the long term results at the present time. Three failure were observed after one course of CHA Promyelo. These 3 patients achieved CR after treatment with high dose Ara-C and Amsacrine. Two relapsed (3 months, 14 months). One has a myelodysplastic syndrome.

Eight patients died during induction. Three of them died before d5 (alveolar hemorrhage : 1 ; leucostasis : 2). The WBC count of these 3 patients (respectively 6.6, 41 and 126 x10^3/mm3) did not change between d1-d3. Three patients died during aplasia (multivisceral failure : 2 ; gastro intestinal bleeding and neurological toxicity of Ara-C : 1). Two patients died from septic shock after CR achievement.

2) Comparison with our first series of M3 patients
When compared to our series of 57 patients treated with conventional therapy (3d./5d) prior to 1982, the CR rate raised from 53 to 72 % (n.s.) (Table 4), and the death rate during induction fell up from 47 to 20 % (p<0.02). However, this improvement of aplasia survival was not clearly associated with a better DIC course during progressive induction, as far as fibrinogen and factor V levels were studied during therapy (d1 - d3 - d5). There was only a trend for a lower incidence of renal and respiratory failure during induction and both these events remained being related to the course of DIC, as in our first series.

Therefore, other factors were studied to explain this lower incidence of death during induction, specially in the management of infection. The management of infections has been always exactly the same in APL and in other AML and the death rate during induction prior to and after 1982 in non M3-AML in our center was exactly the same (15 % vs 16 %) (Table 4). What has changed in terms of death rate in APL (47 % vs 20 %) seems being really specific to APL and likely realted to DIC. The prognostic factors for CR prior to and after 1983 are summarized in Table 5.

TABLE 4 - APL - COMPARISON WITH OTHER FORMS OF AML (AFTER ONE COURSE OF CHEMOTHERAPY)

	1972-1982		1983-1988	
	APL	OTHER AML	APL	OTHER AML
CR	53%*	63%	72%*	65 %
Failure	0%	21%	8%	20%
Death	47%**	16%	20%	15%
ARA-C IV	5 days		10 days	

* N.S.
** p<.01.

TABLE 5 - PROGNOSTIC FACTORS FOR CR IN APL

	1972-1982 (N=57)	1983-1988 (N=39)
Age < 30 Y.	p<.001	NS
Sex	NS	NS
Fever	p<.05	NS
Hb	NS	NS
Platelets	NS	NS
WBC<15,/mm^3	p<.05	NS*
WBC<5,/mm^3	NS	p<.05
DIC	NS	NS

* Only 3 patients had a WBC count > 15,/mm^3

In terms of disease free survival (DFS), the results of CHA Promyelo are significantly better than the first regimen given prior to 1982 (p<0.02)

3) Comparison with conventional CHA and other forms of AML.

When compared to the first 121 patients achieving CR after one course of CHA in non M3-AML, the results obtained with CHA Promyelo in APL patients were not signifcantly different in terms of DFS. However, the timing of relapse seems to be rather different. After conventional CHA, the relapses occurre mainly during the first year. After CHA promyelo, the relapses occurre during the first as during the second year of CR.

DISCUSSION

APL is a very rare disease and it prevents unicentric clinical trials on short term periods. Considerable variations in the rate of CR are reported in the literature for this disease, varying from 16 to 92 % (Figueroa-Casas 1982,

Kantarjian 1986, Sanz 1988, Cunningham) and, despite many reports on APL, several uncertainties remain more than 15 years after the first important paper on the subject (Bernard 1973) : Is heparin necessary for APL induction ? (Goldberg 1987, Hoyle 1988, Kantarjian 1986). What is the best approach for DIC in APL ?. Does APL need a special therapeutic induction different from that given to other AML ?. Is the duration of CR in APL really better than that of other AML ? (Bernard 1973, Cordonnier 1985, Cunningham).

Following our first study, we had been specially alarmed by the high rate (47 %) of death during induction in our center. Many patients seemed to die from the consequences of worsening of DIC under therapy. Since 1983, the use of a progressive induction was associated with a higher CR rate, and overall a lower death rate during induction. However, with this new therapeutical approach, we were waiting for an improvement in the coagulation parameters (Fg and Factor V) during therapy, when compared to our historical group. Because the course of coagulation parameters were not demonstrative for a better control of DIC, we have only indirect arguments (such as lower incidence of renal and respiratory failure during aplasia) to think that DIC has now less tissular consequences. It is also possible that Fg and Factor V are not the good parameters to follow the course of DIC. In any case, we have now to come back and to randomize conventional therapy versus gradual induction to establish the real need of progressive induction in APL.

Secondly, it has to be stressed that progressive induction is certainly not a good approach for hyperleucocytic patients. Among 3 patients with an initial WBC count higher than 15,000/mm^3, one entered CR but the two other patients died on d3 with a daily increasing WBC count during therapy. These patients need conventional therapy with possibly leucopheresis and/or new approaches for DIC.

In conclusion, progressive induction seems to be an interesting approach for non hyperleucocytic APL patients. When compared to an historical group, it was associated, in our experience with an improvement of aplasia survival, which was our main problem in APL prior to 1982. However, because we have not the biological demonstration that the DIC course is less severe with progressive induction than whit conventional therapy, we decided to randomize the trial. Hyperleucocytic patients have to be excluded of this therapeutic approach.

REFERENCES

Bernard, J., Weil, M., Boiron, M., Jacquillat, C., Flandrin, G., Gemon, M.F. (1973) : Acute promyelocytic leukemia : Results of treatment by Daunorubicin. Blood 41, 489-496.

Cohen, L.F., Balow, J.E., Magrath, I.T., Poplack, D.G., Ziegler, J.L. (1980) : Acute tumor lysis syndrome : a review of 37 patients with Burkitt's lymphoma. Am. J. Med. 68, 486-491.

Cordonnier, C., Vernant, J.P., Brun, B, Gouault-Heilman, M., Kuentz, M., Bierling, P., Farcet, J.P., Rodet, M., Duedari, N., Imbert, M., Jouault, H., Mannoni, P., Reyes, F., Dreyfus, B., Rochant, H. (1985) : Acute promyelocytic leukemia in 57 previously untreated patients. Cancer 55, 18-25.

Cunningham, I., Gee, T.S., Reich, L.M., Kempin, S.J., Naval, A.N., Clarkson, B.D. Acute promyelocytic leukemia : treatment results during a decade at Memorial hospital. Blood, in press.

Figueroa-Casas, J., Fradera, J., Velez-Garcia, E., (1982) Acute promyelocytic leukemia (APML). Clinical presentation and evaluation of 38 patients (abstract). Budapest : International Congress ISHISBT, 95.

Goldberg, M.A., Ginsburg, D., Mayer, R.J., Stone, R.M., Maguire, M., Rosenthal, D.S., Antin, J.H. (1987). Is heparin administration necessary during induction chemotherapy for patients with acute promyelocytic leukemia ?. Blood, 69, 187-191.

Hillestad, L.K. (1957) : Acute promyelocytic leukemia. Acta. Med. Scan., 159, 189-194.

Hoyle, C.F., Swirsky, D.M., Freedman, L., Hayhoye, F.G.J. (1988) : Beneficial effect of heparin in the management of patients with APL. Br. J. Haematol., 68, 283-289.

Kantarjian, H.M., Keating, M.J., Walters, R.S., Estey, E.H., McCredie, K.B., Smith, T.L., Dalton, W.T., Cork, A., Trujillo, J.M., Freireich, E.J. (1986) : Acute promyelocytic leukemia : MD Anderson hospital experience Am. J. Med., 80, 789-797.

Sanz, M.A., Jarque, I., Martin, G., Lorenzo, I., Martinez, J., Rafecas, J., Pastor E., Sayas, M.J., Sanz, G., Gomis, F. (1988) : Acute promyelocytic leukemia : therapy results and prognostic factors, Cancer, 61, 7-13.

Vernant, J.P., Leblond, V., Dreyfus, F., Colombat, P., Pesce, A., Troussard, X., Allard, C., Cordonnier, C., Kuentz, M., Karianakis, G., Bierling, P., Rochant, H. (1986) : Results of CHA in adults with acute myeloïd leukemia. IVth International Symposium on therapy of acute Leukemias. Rome.

A clinical trial on the efficacy of leukocyte-depleted blood components in preventing refractoriness to random platelet support : an interim report

P. Rebulla for the Platelet Support Collaborative Group : C. Andreis,
T. Barbui[1], P. Bellavita[2], M. Boeri, V. Carminati[1], N. Greppi, G. Isacchi[3],
L. Lecchi, A.T. Maiolo[4], F. Malagnino[3], F. Mandelli[3], B. Minetti[1], C. Quarti,
D. Riccardi, G. Scudeller[2], G. Sirchia

Centro Trasfusionale e di Immunologia dei Trapianti, Ospedale Policlinico, Milano, [1] Divisione di Ematologia, [2] Centro Trasfusionale, Ospedali Riuniti, Bergamo, [3] Cattedra di Ematologia, Centro Trasfusionale, Università «La Sapienza», Roma, [4] Istituto di Scienze Mediche, Ospedale Policlinico, Milano, Italy

RIASSUNTO

L'alloimmunizzazione contro antigeni del sistema HLA puo' causare refrattarieta' alla trasfusione di piastrine ed esporre i pazienti al rischio di emorragia cerebrale secondaria a piastrinopenia. Tale alloimmunizzazione e' causata principalmente dai leucociti che contaminano gli emocomponenti standard, e che possono essere rimossi mediante semplici tecniche di filtrazione.
Per valutare se l'alloimmunizzazione e la refrattarieta' alla trasfusione di piastrine possono essere prevenute o ridotte mediante l'uso di emocomponenti deprivati di leucociti, abbiamo eseguito uno studio clinico multicentrico nel quale due gruppi di pazienti oncoematologici hanno ricevuto emocomponenti filtrati o emocomponenti standard. Lo studio e' stato impostato in base ad una prevalenza attesa di alloimmunizzazione del 50% nei riceventi di emocomponenti standard (dati della letteratura), e a una riduzione ipotizzata al 25% nei riceventi di emocomponenti deprivati di leucociti. Un'interim analysis condotta sui primi 70 pazienti arruolati non ha prodotto evidenza di una significativa riduzione dell'alloimmunizzazione e della refrattarieta' nei riceventi di emocomponenti deprivati di leucociti. L'alloimmunizzazione e' risultata presente nel 25% dei trattati rispetto al 33% dei controlli; la refrattarieta' e' comparsa in 2 controlli e in nessuno dei pazienti trattati con emocomponenti deprivati di leucociti. Tali dati non permettono di concludere per una uguaglianza dei due trattamenti. Infatti, a seguito di una elevata prevalenza di alloimmunizzazione all'ammissione (17 pazienti su 70) e di altre cause di scarto, il numero di pazienti disponibili per questa analisi e' risultato tale da ridurre a livelli molto bassi la potenza dell' analisi nel dimostrare una differenza significativa fra i due trattamenti. La potenza e' risultata inoltre ulteriormente ridotta da una prevalenza di alloimmunizzazione nei controlli inferiore all'atteso (33% rispetto al 50% ipotizzato). Tali dati, nonche' la revisione di alcuni simili trial clinici riportati nella letteratura, indicano la necessita' di eseguire un trial clinico di dimensioni adeguate per valutare definitivamente vantaggi e svantaggi dell'uso routinario in oncoematologia di emocomponenti deprivati di leucociti. Cio' e' particolarmente rilevante se si considera che nuove metodologie per la prevenzione della refrattarieta' alla trasfusione di piastrine sono in corso di sperimentazione (nuovi filtri al letto del paziente, irradiazione UV). Inoltre e' necessario valutare accuratamente su un'ampia

popolazione di pazienti leucemici la recente osservazione che i leuco citi contaminanti gli emocomponenti possono essere responsabili di u favorevole effetto di "graft versus leucemia" capace di prolungare l durata della remissione.

Keywords: platelet transfusion, alloimmunization, leukocyte-depletion

INTRODUCTION

Red blood cell and platelet transfusion represent a mainstay in th treatment of a number of hematologic diseases. However, a proportio of recipients of standard blood components develop platelet-reactiv alloantibodies which can reduce the efficacy of and even caus refractoriness to random donor platelet support (Schiffer et al. 1976; Howard & Perkins, 1978; Dutcher et al., 1981; Huart et al. 1983). Such antibodies are stimulated mainly by leukocytes whic contaminate standard blood components (Yankee et al., 1969; Claas e al., 1981), and which can be effectively removed by simple an relatively inexpensive filtration procedures (Diepenhorst et al. 1975; Sirchia et al., 1983a). Although it seems rational to try t prevent alloimmunization and refractoriness by transfusing leukocyte depleted blood components (Herzig et al., 1975; Eernisse & Brand 1981), and the results of some clinical trials support this assumptio (Murphy et al., 1986; Andreu et al., 1987; Sniecinski et al., 1988), in one study the difference in the prevalence of alloimmunizatio between recipients of leukocyte-depleted blood components and control did not reach the 5% level of significance (Schiffer et al., 1983).
We performed a multicenter clinical trial to evaluate th effectiveness of leukocyte-depleted blood components in preventin platelet alloimmunization and refractoriness in a group of patient with hematologic malignancies. The aim of this paper is to presen some results of this investigation and to discuss some methodologica problems encountered during the execution of this trial.

MATERIALS AND METHODS

Study design

A prospective randomized clinical trial was started in Milano, Bergamo and Rome in December 1985. The 3 Centers were selected on the basis o voluntary participation. All new patients admitted to the 3 Center with a diagnosis of leukemia or other hematologic malignancy who wer expected to require repeated red blood cell and platelet transfusion were eligible for enrolment into the trial. Noneligible patients wer those reporting more than 3 transfusions before hospital admission. Enrolled patients were stratified for sex and randomized according t random permuted blocks to receive standard or leukocyte-depleted bloo components. A common record form for data collection was used in the Centers. Serial patients' serum samples were collected every 7-10 days, stored at -20 C, and periodically shipped frozen to th Reference Center, where the serological investigations (see below) were performed. At each transfusion, a minimum data set was collected, including date, number and type of blood components transfused, and i the case of platelet transfusion, pre- and post-transfusion (1-h an 24-h) platelet count, and presence or absence of clinical detrimental factors as fever, infection, consumption coagulopathy, splenomegaly, and of therapy with amphotericin B given in the same day (Kulpa et al., 1981). The data analysis was carried out at the Reference Center, where all raw data were processed with a statistical package. Response variables of the trial were 1) 1-h and 24-h posttransfusion platelet increments, 2) development of leukocyte and platelet alloimmunization, and 3) development of refractoriness to random platelet support. Post-transfusion platelet increments were calculated as per cent of expected, according to the following formula (Duquesnoy et al., 1977):

$$\text{Per cent Increment} = \frac{\text{Post - Pre Platelet Count} \times \text{BV} \times 100}{\text{Number of Platelets Transfused} \times 0.67}$$

The patient's blood volume (BV) was calculated according to Nadler et al. (1962). The number of platelets transfused was derived from the quality control program of each transfusion service participating in the trial. The mean number of platelets per concentrate at the 3 Centers was 65, 50 and 70 x 10^6. When filtered products were given, the platelet number per concentrate was reduced by 10 per cent, which represented the mean platelet loss due to routine filtration (Sirchia et al., 1983a).

Alloimmunization was defined as reactivity with more than 10 per cent of the cell panel (see serological investigations). Refractoriness to random donor platelet support was defined as 1-h increments below 20 per cent of expected on 3 or more consecutive occasions, in the absence of clinical detrimental factors. The value of 20 per cent represents a suggested minimum value which should be exceeded in stable recipients transfused with compatible platelets (Filip et al., 1976); this threshold value was confirmed also in our previous experience with leukemic recipients (Sirchia et al, 1983b).

Patient alloimmunization was considered the primary response variable, since the other 2 parameters monitored (platelet count increment and refractoriness) can depend on other conditions in many patients. Therefore the principal comparison concerned the percentages of alloimmunization in the patients treated with leukocyte-depleted blood components and in the control group. The 5% level of significance was accepted as showing evidence of treatment difference. The trial size was determined considering that about 50% of patients were expected to become alloimmunized in the control group (Schiffer et al., 1976), and that the treatment with leukocyte-depleted blood components could halve the percentage of alloimmunization (Schiffer et al., 1983). Given all the above information, we wanted to be 90% sure that, if leuko-poor treatment was able to halve alloimmunization, this would be detected as statistically significant (i.e. we wanted a potency of 90%). The following formula was used to calculate the trial size (Pocock, 1983):

$$N = \frac{p1 \times (100 - p1) + p2 \times (100 - p2)}{(p2 - p1)^2} \times f(\text{alfa}, \text{beta})$$

N = number of cases required on each treatment;
p1 = 50% (percentage of alloimmunization expected in recipients of standard blood components);
p2 = 25% (percentage of alloimmunization in recipients of leukocyte-depleted blood components which we desired to detect as being different from p1);
alfa = 0.05 (the type I error, or the probability of detecting a significant difference when the treatments are equally

effective);
beta = 0.10 (the type II error, or the probability of not detecting a significant difference when there is a difference of magnitude p1-p2);

f(alfa,beta) is a function of alfa and beta, the value of which is 10.5 for alfa = 0.05 and beta = 0.10.

An unadjusted sample size of 74 patients per treatment (total 148) was calculated. The sample size was adjusted for a drop-out rate R of 10% according to Lachin (1981), by multiplying N by the factor $1/(1-R)^2 = 1.23$, to give a total adjusted sample size of 184 patients.
Moreover, it was planned to perform an interim analysis after the enrolment of 70 patients, i.e. the minimum number which would allow the detection of a significant reduction in the prevalence of alloimmunization from 50% (controls) to 25% (recipients of leukocyte-depleted blood components), if this exists. The aim of the interim analysis was to avoid the possibility of depriving hematologic recipients of the benefits of receiving leukocyte-depleted blood components if a significant advantage of this treatment could be demonstrated before the end of the trial.

Patients

The first 70 patients enrolled (from December 1985 to March 1987) were examined in this interim analysis. The 3 Centers (Milano, Bergamo, Rome) contributed 21, 22 and 27 patients, respectively. General data of this patient population are reported in Table 1. Most patients were affected by acute leukemia.

Table 1. General data of the patient population evaluated in the interim analysis.

Type of blood support	Leukocyte-depleted	Standard
No. of patients	32	38
Sex (males/females)	16/16	22/16
Age (yr, median and range)	39 (10-82)	45 (12-81)
Diagnosis: AML	19	23
ALL	10	11
Other	3	4

At the time of data analysis the following protocol violations were identified: 3 patients in the leukocyte-depleted group received a total of 16 non-filtered units of blood components (14 platelet concentrates and 2 red blood cell units) in 3 transfusions; in all cases this was due to emergency. None of these 3 patients developed alloimmunization. In all cases recipients of the control group received standard blood components.
In the evaluation of platelet increments and of refractoriness 11 patients were excluded from analysis for the following reasons: 8 did not receive platelet transfusions, 1 had been enrolled into the trial although noneligible, 2 dropped out during the first week of

treatment. Of a total of 740 platelet transfusions performed, 1-h and 24-h increments were available in 518 (70%) and 484 (65%) occasions, respectively.
In the evaluation of the development of alloimmunization another 28 patients were excluded from analysis: 17 were found already alloimmunized in the serum sample collected at admission, 4 had no serum samples available, 7 had a follow-up of less than 28 days, a period too short to conclude for prevention of alloimmunization (Schiffer et al., 1983).

Blood components

Standard red blood cells and platelet concentrates were prepared according to Slichter and Harker (1976), from 350-450 mL blood donations collected from healthy volunteers. Leukocyte contamination of standard red blood cells and platelet concentrates was 2650 ± 700 and 127 ± 139 million/unit, respectively. Leukocyte-depleted red blood cells and platelet concentrates were prepared as described (Sirchia et al., 1980, 1983a), by filtration through Erypur (Organon Teknika, The Netherlands), and Imugard IG-500 (Terumo, Japan) filters, respectively. Post-filtration leukocyte contamination was determined in all filtered red blood cell and platelet units by counting the leukocytes found in all fields (18 fields) on both sides of a Burker chamber after 1 in 10 dilution in Turk's solution (0.016% violet gentian in 2% acetic acid) of a representative sample of the filtered unit. The total number of leukocytes contaminating the filtered unit (expressed as million/unit) was calculated by multiplying the mean number of leukocytes per count field (= 0.1uL) by the unit net weight in grams, divided by 10. Filtered red blood cells and platelet concentrates contained no detectable leukocytes in 83% and 73% of cases, respectively. In the remaining cases, only units in which less than 5 million leukocytes per unit were counted were given to recipients of the leukocyte-depleted group. This value represents the lower detection limit of the counting method reported above for a red blood cell unit of 250 grams. Indications for platelet transfusion were: bleeding, wet purpura or platelet count below 20,000/uL; for red blood cell transfusion they were hemoglobin levels below 8 g/dL. Standard dosage of platelet transfusion was 1 concentrate per 10 kg of patient's body weight.

Serological Investigations

Patient sera were screened for the presence of lymphocytotoxic (Bodmer, 1978), granulocyte-reactive (Verheugt et al., 1977), and platelet-reactive (von dem Borne et al., 1978) alloantibodies, neat and after 1 in 4 dilution, against lymphocyte, granulocyte and platelet panels selected from 60 blood donors covering all major HLA-A,B specificities. All serological tests were read blindly with appropriate negative, strong positive and weak positive controls. All positive samples showing weak scores of reactivity with less than 20% of the panel were reconfirmed with a different panel on at least 2 occasions. No result discrepancies were found. In general, one sample per month was examined, or at shorter intervals in alloimmunized patients.

Statistical analysis

Percentages of alloimmunization and of refractoriness were compared using the Fisher's exact probability test. The distributions of 1-h and 24-h increments in leukocyte-depleted and control group patients were compared with the Smirnov test (Smirnov, 1939).

RESULTS

1) Platelet count increments and refractoriness.
The distributions of 1-h platelet count increments of recipients of leukocyte-depleted blood components were comparable to those of the recipients of standard products. Median 1-h increments in leukocyte-depleted and in control groups were 39% and 37%, respectively. As expected, a significant difference was found when 1-h platelet count increments of alloimmunized and non-alloimmunized patients were compared. Median 1-h increments in alloimmunized and in non-alloimmunized patients were 30% and 47%, respectively ($p < 0.05$). Platelet count increments at 24-h were proportionally reduced, (median 24-h increments in leukocyte-depleted and in control groups were 26% and 21%, respectively) and they did not differ significantly. Refractoriness to random donor platelet support developed in 2 control patients and in no recipent of leukocyte-depleted products. Due to the low prevalence of refractoriness in control recipients, (which is difficult to evaluate also because of the high prevalence of clinical detrimental factors), we had no possibility to disclose a significant reduction of refractoriness in recipients of leukocyte-depleted blood components.

2) Alloimmunization.
Of the 31 cases available for the evaluation of the development of alloimmunization, 4 in leukocyte-depleted group (25% of 16, 3 males and 1 female) became alloimmunized, compared to 5 in control group (33% of 15, 1 male and 4 females). Each of 2 of the 4 immunized patients in leukocyte-depleted group had received before enrolment 1 standard transfusion (one consisting of 8 platelet concentrates, and the other of 2 red blood cell units); 1 of the 5 immunized cases of control group had received before admission 1 transfusion consisting of 2 red blood cell units, and another had reported at admission 1 previous pregnancy. None of the 4 alloimmunized patients in leukocyte-depleted group received standard blood components in the period between enrolment and development of alloimmunization. Time to development of alloimmunization, number of transfusions and units given before alloimmunization are reported in Table 2. The data analysis of the group of patients without previous blood transfusion and/or pregnancy is reported in Table 3. Both data sets of Tables 2 and 3 indicate that the use of leukocyte-depleted products was not associated with a significant reduction of alloimmunization, neither in the whole patient group, nor in those reporting no previous immunological stimuli like blood transfusion or pregnancy.
The prevalence of alloimmunization with standard products was lower than that found in other trials (Schiffer et al., 1983; Murphy et al., 1986; Sniecinski et al., 1988); however, due to the unexpectedly high number of patients who were found alloimmunized at enrolment, which greatly reduced the number of patients available for the evaluation of development of alloimmunization, and due to the lower-than-expected prevalence of alloimmunization found with standard products, the potency of this interim analysis to detect a statistically significant reduction in the prevalence of alloimmunization in recipients of leukocyte-depleted blood components was very low (less than 50%).

Table 2. Data (mean and range) from patients evaluable for the development of alloimmunization.

Type of blood support	Leukocyte-depleted	Standard
No. of evaluable pts. (M/F)	9/7	6/9
Days of follow-up	218 (55-502)	256 (74-491)
No. of alloimmunized pts.:	4 (25%)	5 (33%)
Time to alloimmunization (d)	42 (20-83)	105 (45-191)
No. of refractory pts.:	0	2
Blood transfusion:		
a) all pts., total:		
* Platelet transfusions:	13 (1-47)	14 (2-62)
* Platelet units:	85 (3-371)	100 (17-440)
* Red cell transfusions:	13 (3-43)	13 (6-25)
* Red cell units:	19 (4-51)	19 (7-40)
b) alloimmunized pts., before alloimmunization:		
* Platelet transfusions:	9 (7-13)	11 (6-20)
* Platelet units:	54 (36-80)	73 (35-149)
* Red cell transfusions:	10 (5-13)	7 (3-10)
* Red cell units:	13 (6-22)	12 (3-19)

Table 3. Data (mean and range) from the evaluable patient population reporting no previous pregnancy and/or blood transfusion.

Type of blood support	Leukocyte-depleted	Standard
No. of evaluable pts.	12	10
Days of follow-up	185 (55-502)	268 (74-491)
No. of alloimmunized pts.:	2 (17%)	3 (30%)
No. of refractory pts.:	0	2
Total blood transfusion:		
* Platelet transfusions:	13 (1-47)	17 (2-62)
* Platelet units:	86 (3-371)	122 (17-440)
* Red cell transfusions:	13 (3-43)	14 (6-25)
* Red cell units:	19 (4-51)	20 (8-40)

All immunized patients' sera, with the exception of 1 case, showed a positive reaction in the lymphocytotoxicity test, alone (5 of 9), or in combination with the platelet- and/or the granulocyte-immunofluorescence test, suggesting that these sera contained anti-HLA antibodies or mixtures of anti-HLA, platelet- and granulocyte-specific antibodies. The only immunized case serum containing no anti-HLA antibodies showed a positive reaction only in the platelet-immunofluorescence test, suggesting that this serum contained platelet specific antibodies.

Alloantibodies disappeared from the patient's serum in 2 of the 4 alloimmunized cases of leukocyte-depleted group, 30 and 183 days after initial detection, and in 1 of the 5 alloimmunized patients of the control group, 126 days after initial detection.

DISCUSSION

This paper reports the results of an interim analysis of a prospective randomized multicenter clinical trial carried out to evaluate if refractoriness to random platelet support can be prevented in hematologic recipients by the routine use of leukocyte-depleted blood components prepared by a simple and relatively inexpensive filtration technique. Unfortunately, this analysis does not yet answer the question addressed with this trial. The main reasons for this are the high prevalence of alloimmunization at admission, which greatly reduced the number of patients available for this analysis, and the low prevalence of alloimmunization developed by recipients of standard blood components, which is lower than that found in the control groups of other recent similar studies. The prevalence of alloimmunization reported by Schiffer et al. (1983), Murphy et al. (1986), and Sniecinski et al. (1988), ranged from 42 to 50% for recipients of standard blood components, compared to 15-20% for recipients of leukocyte-depleted blood components. Our prevalences were 33% (a value similar to that found by Andreu et al. (1987)) and 25%, respectively; this, more than non-supporting the efficacy of leukocyte-depleted blood components in preventing patients' alloimmunization, indicates that even small differences in the procedures for the preparation of blood components, or in patient treatment and evaluation, could play an important role in determining the prevalence of alloimmunization in recipients of standard and leukocyte-depleted blood products. Moreover, this interim analysis showed that, due to our lower-than-expected prevalence of alloimmunization in standard product recipients, the planning of our trial needs to be modified: in fact, in order to maintain the same statistical design defined at the time of trial planning, a total number of about 400 patients must be enrolled.

It is interesting to note that, although a significant difference in the prevalence of alloimmunization was not found, antibodies seemed to disappear more frequently in recipients of leuko-poor blood than in controls (2 of 4 versus 1 of 5 alloimmunized cases, respectively), and that the only 2 refractory patients belonged to the control group. This latter finding, however, is of difficult interpretation, because of the very high prevalence of clinical detrimental factors capable of reducing the efficacy of platelet support in leukemia patients.

Another interesting finding of this analysis was that a significant proportion of our patients (higher than in other studies) reached the hospital already alloimmunized, or recently stimulated by a standard blood transfusion. As already pointed out (Schiffer et al., 1983), this probably reduces the proportion of patients who could potentially

benefit from a leukocyte-depleted blood support.
A series of studies recently appeared in the literature reporting the results of trials performed with the same aim as ours (Schiffer et al., 1983; Murphy et al., 1986; Andreu et al., 1987; Sniecinski et al., 1988). In all these trials the size was small, which precluded the possibility of giving strong evidence in favor of or against a policy for the routine treatment of hematologic recipients with leukocyte-depleted blood components. In fact, in some of these studies, moving just one or two cases from one to another cell of the 2 x 2 contingency table which summarizes the results causes the conventional statistical significance to be lost. Moreover, a small trial size causes also a low potency in detecting a difference, even if it exists. In this regard, it can be calculated that the potency of a trial with 50 evaluable patients per treatment in disclosing a reduction in alloimmunization from 50% to 25% of recipients is about 75%, a value lower than recommended (Friedman et al., 1983). Our trial was not free of the problems related to size, as indicated by the fact that 18 months were necessary to enrol 70 patients, i.e. a minimum number to perform the interim analysis reported here. Therefore, we explored the possibility of performing a meta-analysis of the trials reported in the literature, but unfortunately all trials differ substantially for several aspects, which greatly limits the theoretical possibilities of a meta-analysis.
All these elements point to the conclusion that a large, multicenter, properly designed clinical trial is warranted to definitely evaluate advantages, disadvantages, cost-effectiveness and feasibility of a routine blood support with leukocyte-depleted blood products in hematologic recipients. The reasons for this become even more apparent if it is considered that new and more effective bedside filters for leukocyte removal, as well as other technologies for preventing platelet refractoriness, like UV irradiation, (Slichter et al., 1987), are becoming available; moreover, other potential benefits of leukocyte removal from blood components, including a reduction of transfusion-transmitted viral infections (Verdonck et al., 1985; Murphy et al., 1988a; Riccardi et al., 1988) have not been fully evaluated.
Finally, the claim that leukocytes contaminating blood components can increase the time to relapse in leukemic patients through a "graft versus leukemia" effect (Tucker et al., 1988) should be carefully investigated.

Grant CNR 85.02377.44

ABSTRACT

Alloimmunization to HLA antigens can cause refractoriness to random-donor platelet support in chronic recipients of blood transfusion, and increase the risk of hemorrhage secondary to thrombocytopenia. We performed a clinical trial to evaluate if alloimmunization and refractoriness can be prevented in hematologic patients by using leukocyte-depleted red blood cells and platelet concentrates prepared by simple filtration techniques. The trial design was based on an expected prevalence of alloimmunization of 50 per cent in recipients of standard products, and on a hypothetical reduction of alloimmunization to 25 per cent by the use of leukocyte-depleted blood components. An interim analysis of the first 70 patients enrolled in the trial did not produce evidence of a significant reduction in the prevalence of alloimmunization (25% vs 33% of controls) or refractoriness (0 of 32 cases vs 2 of 38 controls). However, due to the small number of evaluable patients, the potency of this analysis in disclosing a significant reduction of alloimmunization in recipients of leukocyte-depleted blood was very small. Based on these and other data reported in the literature, we believe that a large, multicenter, properly designed clinical trial with a total size of about 400 cases is warranted to definitely assess advantages and disadvantages of a routine policy with leukocyte-depleted blood components in hematologic recipients. This is particularly relevant considering that new techniques are becoming available for the prevention of platelet refractoriness, and that a claim of a potential benefit of contaminating leukocytes in terms of "graft versus leukemia" effect needs to be thoroughly evaluated.

REFERENCES

Andreu, G., Dewailly, J., Leberre, C., Carre, M.C., Paitre, M.L., Fauchet, R., Tardivel, R., Devers, L., Soreau, E., Lam, Y., Boccaccio, C., Piard, N., Genetet, B. (1987): Prevention of HLA immunization with leukocyte-poor packed red cells and platelet concentrates obtained by filtration. Transfusion 27, 512 (abstract).

Bodmer, J.G. (1978): Ia antigens. Definition of the HLA-DRw specificities. Brit. Med. Bull. 34, 233-240.

Borne, A.E.G.Kr. von dem, Verheugt, F.W.A., Riesz, E., von Oosterhof, F., Brutel de la Riviere A., Engelfriet, C.P. (1978): A simple immunofluorescence test for the detection of platelet antibodies. Brit. J. Haematol. 39, 195-207.

Claas, F.H.J., Smeenk, R.J.T., Schmidt, R., van Steenbrugge, J.G., Eernisse, J.G. (1981): Alloimmunization against the MHC antigens after platelet transfusion is due to contaminating leukocytes in the platelet suspension. Exp. Hematol. 9, 84-9.

Diepenhorst, P., Sprokholt, R., Prins, H.K. (1972): Removal of leukocytes from whole blood and erythrocyte suspensions by filtration through cotton wool. I. Filtration technique. Vox Sang. 23, 308-20.

Duquesnoy, R.J., Filip, D.J., Rodey, G.E., Rimm, A.A., Aster, R.H. (1977): Successful transfusion of platelets "mismatched" for HLA antigens to alloimmunized thrombocytopenic patients. Am. J. Hematol. 2, 219-26.

Dutcher, J.P., Schiffer, C.A., Aisner, J., Wiernik, P.H. (1981): Long-term Follow-up of patients with leukemia receiving platelet transfusions: identification of a large group of patients who do not become alloimmunized. Blood 58, 1007-11.

Eernisse, J.G., Brand, A. (1981): Prevention of platelet refractoriness due to HLA antibodies by administration of leukocyte-poor blood components. Exp. Hematol. 9, 77-83.

Filip, D.J., Duquesnoy, R.J., Aster, R.H. (1976): Predictive value of cross-matching for transfusion of platelet concentrates to alloimmunized recipients. Am. J. Hematol. 1, 471-9.

Friedman, L.M., Furberg, C.D., DeMets, D.L. (1985): Fundamentals of clinical trials, 2nd edn, p.92. Littleton (Mass); PSG Publishing Company.

Herzig, R.H., Herzig, G.P., Bull, M.I., Decter, J.A., Lohrmann, H.P., Stout, F.G., Yankee, R.A., Graw, R.G.Jr. (1975): Correction of poor platelet transfusion responses with leukocyte-poor HL-A-matched platelet concentrates. Blood 46, 743-750.

Howard, J.E., Perkins, H.A. (1978): The natural history of alloimmunization to platelets. Transfusion 18, 496-503.
Huart, J.J., Jouet, J.P., Bauters, F., Goudemand, M. (1983): Le traitement des accidents hemorragiques au cours des leucemies aigues et des aplasies medullaires. Nouv. Rev. Fr. Hematol. 25, 229-233.
Kulpa, J., Zaroulis, C.G., Good, R.A., Kutti J. (1981): Altered platelet function and circulation induced by amphotericin B in leukemic patients after platelet transfusion. Transfusion 21, 74-6
Lachin, J.M. (1981): Introduction to sample size determination and power analysis for clinical trials. Controlled Clin. Trials 2, 93-113.
Murphy, M.F., Metcalfe, P., Thomas, H., Eve, J., Ord, J., Lister, T.A., Waters, A.H. (1986): Use of leukocyte-poor blood components and HLA-matched-platelet donors to prevent HLA alloimmunization. Brit. J. Haematol. 62, 529-534.
Murphy, M.F., Grint, P.C.A., Hardiman, A.E., Lister, T.A., Waters, A.H., (1988): Use of leukocyte-poor blood components to prevent primary cytomegalovirus (CMV) infection during remission induction therapy for acute leukaemia. XX Congress of the International Society of Blood Transfusion, London. Book of Abstracts, p. 60.
Nadler, S.B., Hidalgo, J.U., Bloch, T. (1962): Prediction of blood volume in normal human adults. Surgery 5, 224-32.
Pocock, S.J. (1983): Clinical trials: a practical approach, pp 123-41. Chichester: John Wiley & Sons.
Riccardi, D., Rebulla, P., Mozzana, R., Andreis, C., Lambertenghi, G., Mozzi, F., Giovanetti, A.M., Isacchi, G., Barbui, T., Scudeller, G., Sirchia, G. (1988): Blood transfusion complications in bone marrow transplant. XXII Congress of the International Society of Hematology. Milano. Book of Abstracts, p. 90.
Schiffer, C.A., Lichtenfeld, J.L., Wiernik, P.H., Mardiney, M.R., Joseph, J.M. (1976): Antibody response in patients with acute nonlymphocytic leukemia. Cancer 37, 2177-82.
Schiffer, C.A., Dutcher, J.P., Aisner, J., Hogge, D., Wiernik, P.H., Reilly, J.P. (1983): A randomized trial of leukocyte-depleted platelet transfusion to modify alloimmunization in patients with leukemia. Blood 62, 815-820.
Sirchia, G., Parravicini, A., Rebulla. P., Fattori, L., Milani, S. (1980): Evaluation of three procedures for the preparation of leukocyte-poor and leukocyte-free red blood cells for transfusion. Vox Sang. 38, 197-204.
Sirchia, G., Parravicini, A., Rebulla, P., Bertolini, F., Morelati, F., Marconi, M. (1983a): Preparation of leukocyte-free platelets for transfusion by filtration through cotton wool. Vox Sang. 44, 115-120.
Sirchia, G., Rebulla, P., Riccardi, D., Marconi, M., Greppi, N., Maiolo, A.T., Polli, E. (1983b): La trasfusione di piastrine in ematologia: alcuni aspetti critici. Riv. Emoter. Immunoemat. 30, 81-93.
Slichter, S.J., Harker, L.A. (1976): Preparation and storage of platelet concentrates. I. Factors influencing the harvest of viable platelets from whole blood. Brit. J. Haematol. 34, 395-402.
Slichter, S.J., Deeg, H.J., Kennedy, M.S. (1987): Prevention of platelet alloimmunization in dogs with systemic cyclosporine and by UV-irradiation or cyclosporine-loading of donor

platelets. Blood 69, 414-8.
Smirnov, N.V. (1939): Estimate of the deviation between empirical distribution functions in two independent samples. (In Russian.) Bull. Moskow Univ. 2, 3-16.
Sniecinski, I., O'Donnel, M.R., Nowicki, B., Hill, L.R. (1988): Prevention of refractoriness and HLA-alloimmunization using filtered blood products. Blood 71, 1402-7.
Tucker, J., Murphy, M.F., Gregory, W.M., Waters, A.H., Rohatiner, A.Z.S., Lister, T.A. (1988): Removal of graft-versus-leukaemia (GvL) effect by the use of leucocyte-poor blood components in patients with acute myeloblastic leukaemia (AML). Brit. J. Haematol. 69, 118 (abstract).
Verdonck, L.F., Middeldorp, J.M., Kreeft, H.A.J.G., Hauw The, T., Hekker, A., De Gast G.C. (1985): Primary cytomegalovirus infection and its prevention after autologous bone marrow transplantation. Transplantation 39, 455-7.
Verheugt, F.W.A., Borne, A.E.G.Kr. von dem, Decary, F., Engelfriet, C.P. (1977): The detection of granulocyte allo-antibodies with an indirect immunofluorescence test. Brit. J. Haematol. 36, 533-544.
Yankee, R.A., Grumet, F.C., Rogentine, G.N. (1969): Platelet transfusion therapy. The selection of compatible platelet donors for refractory patients by lymphocyte HL-A typing. New Engl. J. Med. 281, 1208-12.

Haemocomponents and alloimmunization in the supportive care of leukemic patients

A. Sagripanti, R. Grazzini*, F. Pecori[1], B. Grassi

Servizio di Ematologia, Clinica Medica I, Università degli Studi di Pisa, and [1] Servizio di Immunoematologia, Spedali Riuniti S. Chiara in Pisa, via Roma, 56100 Pisa, Italy

ABSTRACT

Lymphocytotoxic alloantibodies and antiplatelet alloantibodies were searched in the sera of 57 multitransfused adult patients affected with haematological malignancies. Microlymphocytotoxicity test and platelet suspension indirect immunofluorescence test were performed against comprehensive panels from selected donors; a chloroquine modification of platelet suspension test was also carried out to detect thrombocytic specific antibodies. Eighteen subjects (31%) revealed anti HLA antibodies; one of them had platelet specific antibodies too; the alloantibodies were multispecific in 16 cases. In our patients alloimmunization was an early onset event, unrelated to the amount of units transfused and to the kind of haemocomponent used; alloimmunization rate was higher in acute non lymphoid leukemia and in blast crisis rather than in acute lymphoid leukemia.

KEYWORDS

Alloimmunization, haematological malignancies, refractoriness to blood transfusion, platelet concentrates

INTRODUCTION

Advances in designing aggressive polychemotherapic regimens for leukemic patients have developed in parallel with technological progress in blood transfusion support. The availability of effective platelet transfusion products has decreased mortality from bleeding in leukemic patients; moreover neutropenic patients with overwhelming infections might benefit by granulocyte concentrates. Unfortunately refractoriness occurs in many multitransfused subjects; immunological factors as well as other causes (hypersplenism, sepsis, intravascular coagulation, bleeding etc.) may account for poor response to transfusion. Aim of the study is to determine the alloimmunization rate to random donor transfusions in various haematological malignancies and to characterize time of onset, antigen specificity and pattern of disappearance of the alloantibodies involved.

MATERIAL AND METHODS

Patients
We have studied 57 patients, 30 males and 27 females, aged 15 to 78 years, who received haemocomponents for at least 5 days. Transfused units (platelet concentrates, granulocyte concentrates and/or packed red cells) ranged from 5 to 72 (mean 14 units). There were 18 cases of acute non lymphocytic leukemia, 6 acute lymphocytic leukemia, 7 blastic phase of chronic myelogenous leukemia, 4 myelodysplastic syndromes, 10 agnogenic myeloid metaplasia, 12 non-Hodgkin lymphoma. All the leukemic patients received polychemotherapy according to current schemes.

Haemocomponents
Packed red cells were prepared without leukocyte removing procedure and were administered when hemoglobin level was below 6-8 g/dL.
Platelet and granulocyte concentrates were obtained from single random donors by apheresis using discontinous flow cell separators (DIDECO BT 740). Platelets were transfused prophylactically when platelet count dropped below 15×10^9/L and therapeutically in decompensated intravascular coagulation syndrome as well as in major bleeding events. Granulocytes were administered therapeutically to neutropenic patients (granulocyte count $< 0.5 \times 10^9$/L) presenting persistent high fever (>39°C) unresponsive to antibiotics for at least 3 days.

Laboratory tests
Serum samples from each patient were screened for alloantibodies basally and then 3 weeks after every transfusional treatment. The following techniques were used:
1. Microlymphocytotoxicity test (LCT) according to Terasaki (Mittal, 1978).
2. Platelet suspension indirect immunofluorescence test (PSIFT) according to Von Dem Borne (1978).
3. A chloroquine modification of PSIFT according to Metcalfe (Norhagen, 1985).

Lymphocytotoxic antibodies were tested against a comprehensive HLA-typed lymphocyte panel from 20 selected donors, covering all major HLA A,B specificities. The test was considered positive if more than 50% lymphocytes from one or more donors were killed. The alloantibody was defined monospecific if serum sample reacted with only one antigen specificity and multispecific if serum sample reacted with the majority of donor cells.
Antiplatelet antibodies were tested against a comprehensive platelet panel from 10 0-group donors known to contain the main thrombocyte specific antigens. When a subject was positive for PSIFT, a chloroquine modification of PSIFT was also carried out in order to detect the presence of non HLA platelet specific antibodies. Indeed chloroquine-treated platelets loss their HLA antigens, but mantain thrombocytic specific antigens, that are more tightly bound to cell membrane

RESULTS

Serum alloantibodies were detected in 18 out 57 patients (31%), 10 males and 8 females. All the 18 subjects had a positive LCT and simultaneously a positive PSIFT; only one of them had also a positive chloroquine test. As it concerns the incidence of alloimmunization in the various haematological malignancies, 9/18 cases of acute non lymphocytic leukemia, 5/7 cases of blastic phase of chronic myelogenous leukemia, 1/4 cases of myelodysplastic syndromes, 1/10 cases of agnogenic myeloid metaplasia and 2/12 cases of non-Hodgkin lymphoma were positive for alloantibodies.

In 17 patients sera reacted with the majority of donor samples in the panel, indicating the presence of multispecific antibodies. Only one patient exhibited a monospecific alloantibody, reacting with the A3 antigen of HLA system.
We have not found any significant correlation between tha number of transfused units and the frequency of alloimmunization. Furthemore there was no relationship between the type of haemocomponent administrated (packed red cells versus platelet and granulocyte concentrates) and the alloimmunization rate; indeed 8 patients became sensitized after being transfused with only packed red cells.
As it concerns the chronological pattern of the immune response, all the patients developed alloantibodies a few weeks (median 2.6 weeks) after the beginning of transfusional support. Serial determinations of serum samples in patients who had a positive test showed the persistence of alloimmunization even after the suspension of blood transfusion. On the other hand the subjects who were negative for serum alloantibodies after the first 10 days of blood support did not develop sensitivization afterwards.
Nine out of 18 immunized patients (50%) manifested one or more transfusion reactions (chills and hypertermia) in the course of haemocomponent administration; on the other side only 2 out 29 subjects who were negative for alloantibodies (7%) exhibited typical transfusion reactions.

DISCUSSION

The simultaneous positivity of LCT and PSIFT in our subjects suggest the presence of HLA specific alloantibodies; this indicates a major role for HLA system in the immune response to blood products, in agreement with previous reports.
Only one patient of ours had also evidence of platelet specific alloantibodies; the occurrence of non HLA thrombocytic specific antibodies is a rather infrequent, though not rare, complication, that may account for refractoriness to HLA-matched platelets.
The alloimmunization rate we have found is somewhat lower in comparison to the findings of other authors; really the use of single donor platelet concentrates in our series may account for the difference. We point out the high incidence of sensitization during the blastic phase of chronic myelogenous leukemia. Although all the patients affected with acute lymphocytic leukemia were treated by antiblastic myelosuppressive agents, none of them did form antibodies: we suppose that patients with acute lymphocytic leukemia are less prone to alloimmunization for causes inherent to their disease itself; alternatively high dose corticosteroids, administered in current regimens, might interfere with immune regulatory mechanisms.
The transfusion of packed red cells, without leukoplatelet concentrates, elicited an anti HLA immune response in a considerable number of our patients: leukocytes and platelets, present in routinely prepared red cell concentrates, as well as HLA antigens expressed in reticulocytes, may account for anti HLA sensitization.
In our series alloimmunization developed in an early stage of the transfusional treatment; once immunization has occurred, it persisted in spite of suspension of blood support. On the other hand an appreciable number of patients failed to form antibodies in spite of heavy transfusional treatment. Taken as a whole, these findings suggest that a genetic predisposition may regulate the immune response, once a sufficient exposure to blood antigens has occurred.
The presence of alloantibodies significantly correlated with the occurrence of transfusion reactions, pointing out a pathogenetic role for alloantibodies.

CONCLUSIONS

Alloimmunization is a rather common early-onset event in multitransfused patients affected with haematological malignancies, partucularly in acute non lymphoid leukemia and in blastic crisis of chronic myelogenous leukemia; HLA A,B antigens, that are present both in leukocytes and in platelets, seem to play a major role in alloimmune response. Administration of leukocyte-depleted blood products has been advocated to reduce the frequency of alloimmunization, but results has been questionable (NIHCC, 1987). Once sensitization has occurred, the trasfusion of cross matched platelets or granulocytes appears to be feasible and effective, expecially in patients who experienced refractoriness and severe reactions.

SUMMARY

Aim of the study is to determine the frequency of alloimmunization in multitransfused haematological patients and to characterize time of onset, antigen specificity and pattern of disappearance of alloantibodies. Fifty-seven adult patients (22 with acute non lymphoid leukemia or myelodysplastic syndrome, 6 with acute lymphoid leukemia, 10 with agnogenic myeloid metaplasia, 7 with blastic crisis of chronic myeloid leukemia and 12 with non-Hodgkin lymphoma), who received packed red cells and/or leukoplatelet concentrates, were examined for serum alloantibodies. Antilymphocyte antibodies (microlymphocytotoxicity test) were detected in 18 subjects: 9 of them had acute non lymphoid leukemia and 5 were in blastic crisis. Antiplatelet antibodies (indirect immunofluorescence test) were detected in 18 subjects, who were the same positive for lymphocytotoxic antibodies. Alloimmunization developed at an early stage of transfusional treatment and persisted after suspension of blood support; it was unrelated to the amount of units transfused and to the kind of haemocomponent; the patients who were negative after the first 10 transfusions did not sensitized afterwards. A chloroquine modification of the fluorescent antiglobulin technique was carried out in the 18 positive patients; only one of them had a positive result.

REFERENCES

Borne,A.E.G.von dem et al.(1978): A simple immunofluorescence test for the detection of platelet antibodies. Br.J.Haematol.,39, 195-207.
Mittal,K.K.(1978): Workshop report: standardization of the HLA-typing method and reagents. Vox Sang.34, 58-63.
National Institutes of Health Consensus Conference: Platelet Transfusion Therapy. Transfusion Medicine Reviews (1987) 1, 195-200.
Norhagen,R., Flaathen,S.T.(1985): Chloroquine removal of HLA antigens from platelets for the platelet immunofluorescence test. Vox Sang.48, 156-159.

Blood products for the support of bone marrow transplantation

C. Giardini, F. Agostinelli, M. Galimberti, P. Polchi, P. Politi, F. Manenti, S.M.T. Durazzi, C. Rossi, D. Baronciani, G. Lucarelli

Division of Hematology, Bone Marrow Transplantation Center, Pesaro Hospital, Italy

SUMMARY:
Marrow graft recipients require extensive transfusions after transplantation, particularly during the period of severe bone marrow aplasia. Significant risk factors associated with increased support necessity in our patients have been:
- R.B.C. support: severe splenomegaly, ABO-incompatible marrow donors, severe Ac.GVHD, hemorrhagic cystitis;
- Platelet support: severe splenomegaly, severe Ac. GVHD, hemorrhagic cystitis.
Alloimmunization and risk of transmission of ubiquitous viruses by blood components (like Cytomegalovirus and Epstein-Barr) remain open problems in the transfusion therapy of transplanted patients.

Allogeneic bone marrow transplantation (B.M.T.) has been used with increasing success for the treatment of various malignant and hereditary hematological disorders. Because of the prolonged period of severe bone marrow aplasia following the conditioning regimen, intensive substitution of blood components is essential during this period.

BLOOD TRANSFUSION IN THE PRE-TRANSPLANT PERIOD.

Before grafting almost all marrow transplant candidates go through periods of marrow failure either due to their disease or its treatment with chemotherapeutic agents:
patients with Chronic Myeloid Leukemia (C.M.L.) usually do not need any transfusion therapy during the course of their disease, while in Chronic Phase. However, patients with Acute Leukemia (A.L.) during chemotherapy, patients with Aplastic anemia (A.A.) and, obviously, patients with homozygous hemoglobinopathies like ß-major thalassemia, undergo transfusion support before transplantation. For these patients the avoidence of alloimmunization is of primary importance.

HLA antigens:

Immunization for the major transplantation antigens is a two-signal process in which stimulation of helper T cells is mainly induced by a class-II antigen transfused into marrow graft recipients should be irradiated to prevent the proliferation of lymphoid cells.

In a series of transplanted patients reported by Storb, patients with Acute Leykemia (A.L.) in relapse required a higher number of R.B.C. and platelet transfusions compared with patients with A.L. in remission; also patients with A.A. had support requirement comparable with patients with A.L. in relapse. For patients with C.M.L., those who were in Blast crisis at time of transplant needed an intensive support therapy compared with patients in Chronic phase.

In a series of 189 consecutive patients transplanted in our division for ß-major thalassemia, the mean value of transfusion units has been 4.9 for each patient. Factor of risk associated with an increased support requiremenr were:
- severe splenomegaly (more than 3 cm);
- ABO incompatible marrow donors;
- Acute GVHD grade III-IV;
- hemorrhagic cystitis.

Patients with previous splenectomy seem to require a smaller number of transfusion units (P: N.S.).

TABLE I: TRANSFUSION SUPPORT.

	PATIENTS	R.B.C.(MEAN)	P
TOTAL	189	4.9	
SEVERE SPLENOMEGALY (> 3cm)	36	8.6	>0.001
ABO-INCOMPATIBLE MARROW DONORS	65	6.5	<0.05
SEVERE Ac. GVHD (III-IV)	28	10.07	<0.001
HEMORRHAGIC CYSTITIS	33	7.3	<0.001
PREVIOUS SPLENECTOMY	34	3.7	N.S.

No significant difference has been seen between patients who received less than one hundred transfusions pre-transplant and patients who received over one hundred units (P: bordeline).

Platelet transfusions:

multiple platelet support from single donors is necessary to maintain platelet blood levels higher than 20,000 per cubic millimeter, to avoid risk of untreatable spontaneous bleeding.

Patients with high fever, disseminated infections, hemorrhage, severe Ac. GVHD or previous sensitization to platelet-surface antigens, need intensive platelet support. HLA non-identical family donors or random donors are generally used. The marrow donor or other HLA-identical family donors (when available) are used to avoid risk of allo-immunization. All platelet bags must be screened for hepatitis markers, HIV, CMV. The range of platelet bag count has been between 0.5 and 3 x 10^{11} platelets per unit in our experience. In our series of patients (TABLE II) the mean value of platelet units has been 11 for each patient. Patients with severe splenomegaly, severe Ac.GVHD and hemorrhagic cystitis have a significantly higher need for platelet support. On the contrary, patients with

difference as measured in vitro by the mixed lymphocyte culture reaction.
In the effector phase, cytotoxic cells and/or antibodies against class-I and class-II antigens can be detected.
In the peripheral blood class-II antigens are mainly expressed on B lymphocytes and monocytes and the approach to minimize HLA sensitization is based on leucocyte depletion of the various blood components.
Leucocyte depletion of red blood cell (RBC) transfusions can be obtained by filtration; leucocyte depletion of platelets can be obtained by an extra step centrifugation or by filtration (as proposed by Sirchia).
Transfusions of blood products from family donors should be avoided prior to transplantation, because of possible sensitization to non-HLA antigens.

Transfusions before marrow transplantation in patients with Aplastic Anemia:

Patients with A.A. are immunologically competent and, thus, more likely to become sensitized to histocompatibility antigens.
A series of clinical trials has shown that patients with A.A. submitted to transfusion support before transplant have an increased rejection rate and a decreased survival compared with untransfused patients.
For this reason it is important for the physician to be aware of the possibility of marrow transplantation when a patient with aplastic anemia is first diagnosed.
HLA typing of patient and all family members should be done immediately at diagnosis and, if an HLA-identical family member is identified, early transplantation must be considered as first-line therapy.
In that case, transfusions of blood products should not be given unless indicated by urgent medical necessity; transfusions from family members should not be given in any case.

BLOOD TRANSFUSION AFTER MARROW TRANSPLANTATION.

After grafting there is a period of pancytopenia lasting 14-30 days before graft function appears.
Effective support with blood products during this period of marrow failure is essential to achieve success in marrow transplantation.
Therefore we will attempt to discuss the principles governing trasfusion support of various blood components.

Red Blood cell transfusions:

The aim is to maintain a hemoglobin level higher than 8-9 gr.% or HcT higher than 20-25%.
Patients with high fever, disseminated infections, hemorrhage or V.O.D. need an intensive support therapy.
Patients generally require R.B.C. support for 6-12 weeks until graft erythropoiesis is adequate, although most transfusions are required within the first 4 weeks of transplantation.
In our experience, leucocyte-poor preparations are necessary for support of polytransfused patients, to avoid reactions like chills and fever.
Viable lymphocytes capable of causing GVHD in severely immunosuppressed patients are present in all cellular transfusion products; therefore, all blood products

previous splenectomy seem to require a smaller number of platelet units (P:N.S.).

TABLE II: PLATELET SUPPORT.

	PATIENTS	PLATELET BAGS (MEAN)	P
TOTAL	189	11	
SEVERE SPLENOMEGALY (>3 cm.)	36	17.1	<0.001
SEVERE Ac. GVHD (III-IV)	29	19.0	<0.001
HEMORRHAGIC CYSTITIS	33	15.5	<0.05
PREVIOUS SPLENECTOMY	32	8.3	N.S.

Granulocyte transfusions:

To date, there is no consensus in the literature about the indications for granulocyte transfusions in transplanted patients; in fact the effectiveness of this treatment is uncertain and there is a high risk of transfusion-related complications, such as fever, dyspnea, pulmonary complications, CMV infections. In a series of 19 patients transplanted in our division for end-stage leukemia who received granulocyte transfusions during the aplastic period, compared with 26 patients in the control Group, we observed:
-a higher rate of septicemia resolution (64% versus 28%: P:N.S.);
-a higher rate of resolution of localized infections (36% versus 11%: P:N.S.);
but no difference in mortality in the two Groups.
For this reason, considering the severe adverse reactions often observed during infusion, we have ceased to use granulocyte transfusions in transplanted patients.

Plasma and protein transfusions:

Intravenous immunoglobulin administration has been included in our transplant protocol to enhance prophylaxis against infections; also in this case, the therapy has certain drawbacks, such as its high cost, the fact that it can give rise to adverse reactions, and that its effectiveness is not certain.
In patients with severe Ac. GVHD, especially of the gastrointestinal tract, a large amount of albumin and plasma support may be necessary because of protein-losing enteropathy, increased vascular permeability, and the catabolic condition of the patient.

REFERENCES.

Brand, A. (1984): Blood component therapy in Bone Marrow Transplantation.
    Seminars in Hematology, 20, 2, 141-155.
Schiffer, C.A. (1982): Platelet transfusions from single donors. The New England
    Journal of Medicine, 307, 4, 245-247.
Storb, R. (1981): Transfusion problems associated with transplantation.
    Seminars in Hematology, 18, 2, 163-176.

Isolator lysis-centrifugation blood culture tube analysis in a series of granulocytopenic leukemic patients

A. Bosi, R. Fanci, A. Orsi[1], P. Pecile[1], P. Rossi Ferrini

Cattedra e Divisione di Ematologia and [1] Laboratorio di Batteriologia e Virologia
Università degli Studi ed Ospedale di Careggi, I-50134, Firenze, Italy

SUMMARY

An analysis of blood cultures in patients with acute leukemia in aplastic phase following to antineoplastic regimen, is reported. In 20 from 50 cultures (40%) the tube showed a bacterial infection. The isolated organisms were gram negative rods in 75% of cultures and gram positive in 25%. The identified gram negative organisms were Enterobacteriaceae in 50% of samples, Pseudomonadaceae in 25%: Ps aeruginosa 10% and Pseudomonas spp 15% ; the gram positive rods were Staphylococcus coagulase negative in 10%, Staphylococcus aureus in 10%, Streptococcus alpha- haemoliticus in 5%. Anaerobic organisms were not detected. These findings confirm the role of gram negative bacilli in the pathogenesis of infections. Moreover the emerging role of gram positive organisms should be stressed.

KEYWORDS

Isolator, blood cultures, acute leukemia, infections, gram negative bacilli.

INTRODUCTION

Bacterial infections and sepsis occur more frequently when the absolute neutrophil count falls under $1 \times 10^9/1$ (Bodey, 1966). In this patient group the clinical course of infections is very poor and often fatal. When the results of bacteriological cultures are available, frequently the patient's status is already compromised. So the a-priori knowledge of the organisms more frequently identified in the same set of patients in a nosocomial environment is very helpful in employing an empiric antibiotic protocol (Pizzo, 1985; Verhagen, 1987). In this paper we report an analysis of blood cultures in patients with acute leukemia in aplastic phase sequent to antineoplastic regimen observed at the Division of hematology of the University of Florence. Blood cultures were performed with the Isolator lysis-centrifugation blood culture tube (Du Pont Co.), a methodology that offered a significant improvement over an unvented broth bottle or a vented biphasic bottle for the detection of septicemia due to certain microrganism (Henry, 1983).

PATIENTS AND METHODS

From January to December 1987, 31 patients with acute leukemia in aplastic phase after induction chemotherapy were evaluated at the Division of Hematology of the University of Florence, Italy, for analysis of blood cultures. All patients were subjected to prophylactic measures. Patients were isolated in a protected environment and treated with decontamination procedures as skin cleansing and mucocutaneous decontamination with clorexidine gluconate washings; oral non-absorbable antibiotics and antimicotics and trimetoprim/sulfamethoxazole were given. In febrile episodes (fever higher than 38 C and unrelated to transfusions), Isolator lysis-centrifugation blood culture was performed (Henry, 1983; Thomson, 1984). Blood cultures were routinely obtained from peripheral vein. Single blood culture isolates of Gram-positive cocci were considered positive except for Staphylococcus epidermidis which required at least two different positive blood cultures drawn from separate venipuncture sites.

RESULTS

The granulocytopenic episodes observed were 64. In most cases (49), granulocytopenia was very severe (granulocytes <0.2 x 10^9/l) with a total of 1013 days at risk. In 10 cases granulocytes were 0.2 - 0.5 x 10^9/l with overall days at risk of 170 and finally, in 5 cases only, granulocytes were 0.5 - 1 x 10^9/l with overall days at risk of 65. In the 64 episodes overall days at risk of infection were 1248. 49 febrile episodes were observed in 64 granulocytopenic episodes (76.6%); the days with fever were 331 in 1248 days at risk (26.5%). From 50 cultures performed, in 20 (40%) the tube showed a bacterial infection. The isolated organisms are detailed in Table 1.

DISCUSSION

In spite of prophylactic measures, febrile episodes remain a major problem for granulocytopenic patients hospitalized in a conventional environment and were in fact observed in 76.6% of cases in our study. However in our experience the observed ratio of days with fever and days at risk was only 26.5%. In febrile episodes the percentage of positive blood cultures was 40% and Isolator lysis-centrifugation blood culture tube has offered a significant improvement for the detection of bacteria and fungi (Henry, 1983). Our experience confirms the role of gram negative bacilli in the pathogenesis of infections in hospitalized leukemic patients (75%). Moreover, as reported by others (Klestersky, 1986; Valls, 1987; Menichetti, 1988), our findings emphasize the emerging role of gram positive organisms as streptococci and staphylococci (25%). The detection in blood cultures of new gram negative bacilli belonging to the family of Pseudomonadaceae (Ps stutzeri, vesicularis, acidovorans), stresses the need for a strict control program on all hospital personnel and environment as measures for preventing nosocomial infections.

Table 1.   Analysis of blood cultures (Isolator)

	N	%
cultures performed	50	
positive cultures	20	40
gram negative rods	15	75
gram positive rods	5	25
Enterobacteriaceae	10	50
E. Coli	7	35
K. Pneumoniae	1	5
K. Oxytocica	1	5
C. Freundii	1	5
Pseudomonadaceae	5	25
Ps aeruginosa	2	10
Ps vesicularis	1	5
Ps stutzeri	1	5
Ps acidovorans	1	5
Staphylococcus coagulase negative	2	10
Staphylococcus aureus	2	10
Streptococcus alpha-haemoliticus	1	5

REFERENCES

Bodey, G.P. (1966): Quantitative relationships between circulating leukocytes and infections in patients with acute leukemia. Ann. Int. Med. 64, 328-35

Henry, N. K. (1983): Microbiological and clinical evaluation of the Isolator lysis-centrifugation blood culture tube. J. Clin. Microbiol. 17, 864-869.

Klestersky, J. (1986): Concept of empiric therapy with antibiotic combinations. Indications and limits. Am. J. Med. 80, 2-12.

Menichetti, F. (1988): Teicoplanin in empirical combined antibiotic therapy of bacteraemias in bone marrow transplant patients. J. Antimicrob. Chemother. 21, 105-111.

Pizzo, A. (1986): A randomized trial comparing ceftazidime alone with combination antibiotic therapy in cancer patients with fever and neutropenia. N. Engl. J. Med. 315, 552-558.

Thomson, R.B. (1984): Contamination of cultures processed with the Isolator lysis-centrifugation blood culture tube. J. Clin. Microb. 19, 97-99.

Valls, A. (1987): Microorganismos aislados en 54 pacientes sometidos a trasplante de medula osea y valoracion de su sensibilidad a los antimicrobianos. Med. Clin. (Barc) 89, 768-772.

Verhagen, C.S. (1987): Randomized prospective study of ceftazidime versus ceftazidime plus cephalothin in empiric treatment of febrile episodes in severely neutropenic patients. Antimicrob. Agents Chemother. 31, 191-196.

Possible mechanisms of late infections in T-depleted bone marrow transplantation : Ig isotype switches leading to selective IgG2-IgG4 subclass deficiency

A. Velardi, S. Cucciaioni, E. Cimignoli, R. Felicini, N. Albi, C. Dembech, A. Terenzi, F. Grignani, M.F. Martelli

Department of Medicine and¹ Division of Hematology, University of Perugia, Italy

SUMMARY

We report the results of a series of studies aimed at the identification of the mechanisms governing the post-grafting immune recovery process. In this studies, the recovering humoral immune system recapitulates with striking accuracy some of the developmental steps known to occur during human ontogeny. The last maturational step to be observed in this sequence was a selective IgG2 subclass deficiency in all of the long term graft recipients examined which may be relevant to the late bacterial infections known to occur in these patients.

KEY WORDS

BMT, IgG subclass deficiency, bacterial infections

INTRODUCTION

The recovery period which follows allogeneic bone marrow transplantation is known to be associated with a prolonged cellular and humoral immune deficiency syndrome with increased susceptibility to a variety of viral, bacterial, protozoan and fungal pathogens. Granulocytopenia is a cause of infection only limited to the initial 2-3 post-grafting weeks. Afterwards and throughout the ensuing 3-4 months, successfully engrafted recipients may experience a life threatening interstitial pneumonia tipically associated with Pneumocystis Carinii or Cytomegalovirus infection. Hypogammaglobulinemia and B and T-cell functional abnormalities have consistently been reported in this period (Reviewed by: Lum, 1987). T-cell abnormalities comprise inverted T-helper/T-suppressor cell ratios, defective proliferative responses against mitogens or alloantigens, defective helper function for B-cell differentiation, poor IL-2 production and defective generation of cytolytic effector cells in MLR. Rather unexpectedly, immunologically reconstituted healthy long-term survivors (>7 months post-grafting) may continue to exhibit an increased susceptibility to infections mainly caused by Gram+ cocci such as Pneumococcus and impaired antibody responses against bacterial polysaccharide antigens (Atkinson et al., 1979; Winston et al., 1979). It is, therefore, evident that in spite of the identification of such a variety of immunological abnormalities, the real mechanisms underlying the whole post-grafting immune recovery process are largely unknown. It is also not known whether such impaired immune competence plays any role at all with regard to the risk of post-grafting leukemia relapses.

Here we report the results of a series of studies recently performed in our laboratories in order to acquire information on the mechanisms governing the post-grafting immune recovery process. In this studies, the recovering humoral immune system has been investigated against the developmental scheme offered by normal human B-cell ontogeny (Reviwed by: Cooper, 1987). This allowed us to identify a maturational sequence in the post-grafting B-cell recovery process which recapitulates with striking accuracy some of the developmental steps known to occur during human ontogeny. The last maturational step to be observed in this sequence was a selective IgG2 subclass deficiency in all of the long term graft recipients examined which may be relevant to the late bacterial infections known to occur in these patients.

SUBJECTS AND METHODS

The patient population consisted of 10 subjects who underwent allogeneic bone marrow transplantation for hematologic malignancies. The patients (in remission) were prepared for transplantation by cytoreduction according to the protocol of O'Reilly et al. with modifications. The marrow donors were HLA-identical, mixed lymphocyte culture-compatible adult individuals.
The marrow transplants were depleted of T cells (to prevent Graft-versus-Host-Disease) by sequential soybean agglutination and E-rosetting. Phenotypic analyses of B-cell populations was performed by two-color immunofluorescence utilizing antibodies directed against IgM, IgG, IgA, C3d/EBV receptor and CD38 (T10 antigen). T-cell subsets were identified with antibodies directed against CD4, CD8, Leu 7 and CD11b. Analysis of the distribution of the four IgG subclasses amongst bone marrow or in vitro generated plasma cells was performed by two-color immunofluorescence utilizing subclass-specific monoclonal antibodies in combination with anti total IgG antibodies. Serum IgG subclass analyses were performed by radial immunodiffusion.

RESULTS

Two-color immunofluorescence analysis of the recovering B cells after BMT revealed that only 51±8% expressed detectable C3d/EBV receptors, whereas as many as 78±6% expressed CD38 (T10 antigen) (Table 1). In contrast, normal control B cells were >95% C3d/EBV-receptor-positive and <15% CD38-positive. Thus, B cells recovering after BMT exhibited the immature Cd3/EBV-receptor-negative/CD38-positive phenotype, which is typical of fetal B cells (reviewed in ref. 3). Moreover, >95% IgA B cells co-expressed IgM and, to a lesser extent, IgD. Likewise, >95% IgG B cells co-expressed IgM and >80% co-expressed IgD. In contrast, control individuals exhibited very low proportions of IgA or IgG B cells co-expressing IgM or IgD. Therefore, similarly to that observed during human ontogeny, post-grafting IgA and IgG B cells appeared to be recent isotype-switched cells from IgM±IgD (reviewed in Cooper, 1987). We next determined the pattern of acquisition of IgG plasma-cell precursors belonging to each of the four subclasses made available in our marrow graft recipients as a result of the isotype switch process.

Terminal differentiation of plasma cells sinthesising each of the four subclasses is an uneven process in ontogeny and is related to the order of Ig costant region genes on chromosome 14, which is gamma 3, gamma 1, gamma 2, gamma 4 (reviewed in Cooper, 1987). As a consequence, IgG1 and IgG3 levels are relatively higher at birth as opposed to IgG2 and IgG4 which attain adult proportions in late childhood. In our control individuals, the expression of IgG subclasses among PWM-induced IgG plasma cells was comparable to that observed in bone marrow: IgG1≈60%, IgG2≈30%, IgG3≈6%, IgG4≈4%. In striking contrast, marrow graft-recipients exhibited almost undetectable proportions of IgG2 and IgG4 plasma cells both in culture and in bone marrow aspirates up to one year post-grafting. Finally, serum IgG subclass analyses revealed markedly depressed IgG2 and IgG4 levels in all graft recipients examined up to 18 months post-grafting.

Table 1   B-CELL RECONSTITUTION AFTER BMT

a) "B-cell exhibiting immature phenotypes"

	PATIENTS	CONTROLS
% B cells co-expressing, C3d/EBV-receptors:	51±8	96±1*
CD38 (T10 antigen):	78±6	15±2*

b) "Recently isotype-switched B cells co-expressing multiple surface Ig"

	PATIENTS	CONTROLS
% IgA+ B cells co-expressing IgM/IgD:	95±1/85±1	5±1/4±1*
% IgG+ B cells co-expressing IgM/IgD:	96±2/86±2	2±1/2±1*

c) "Uneven emergence of IgG subclasses"

Serum IgG subclasses 7-18 months post-BMT (mg/dl)

	IgG1	IgG2	IgG3	IgG4
PATIENTS:	900±9	80±2	91±2	5±1
CONTROLS:	500±3*	250±2*	50±2*	35±2*

* $P<0.05$

DISCUSSION

The present series of experiments was conducted with the primary aim of acquiring information with regard to the immunodeficiency syndrome which develops following allogeneic bone marrow transplantation. Indeed, in spite of the vast literature describing a variety of post-grafting immunological abnormalities (Reviewed by: Lum, 1987), the mechanisms governing the immune recovery process after BMT are largely unknown.

Our data identify an unprecedented maturational sequence in the post-grafting B-cell recovery process which recapitulates with striking accuracy some of the developmental steps known to occur during human ontogeny (Reviewed by: Cooper, 1987). The last maturational step to be observed in this sequence was a selective IgG2 subclass deficiency in all long term graft recipients examined. Antibody responses against capsular carbohydrate components of Gram+ bacteria are largely contained within the IgG2 subclass of immunoglobulins. As a consequence, our present finding of markedly depressed serum IgG2 levels in long-term marrow graft-recipients may be relevant to the pathogenesis of the late bacterial infections described after BMT (Atkinson et al., 1979; Winston et al., 1979).

RESUME

Dans cette étude nous avons démontré que la reconstitution immunologique après la greffe de moelle osseuse allogenique récapitule certaines étapes du développment documentés pendant l'ontogenèse humaine. Le dernier stade de maturation observé a été un déficit selectiv de la souclasse IgG2 chez tous les survivants a long terme. Cette situation semblent intéressante en relation aux infection bactériennes tardives observées chez ces sujets.

REFERENCES

Atkinson K., R. Storb, R.L. Prentice, P.L. Weiden, R.P. Witherspoon, K. Sullivan, and E.D. Thomas.(1979): Analysis of late infections in 89 long-term survivors of bone marrow transplantation. Blood 53:720-731

Cooper MD.(1987): B lymphocytes. Normal development and function. N Engl J Med 317:1452-1456

Lum LG.(1987): The kinetics of immune reconstitution after human marrow transplantation. Blood 69:369-380

Umetsu D.T., D.M. Ambrosino, I. Quinti, G.R. Siber and R.S. Geha. (1985): Recurrent sinopulmonary infection and impaired antibody response to bacterial capsular polysaccharide antigen in children with selective IgG-subclass deficiency. N Eng J Med 313:1247-1251

Winston D.J., G. Schiffman, D.C. Wang, S.A. Faig, C. Lin, E.L. Marso, W.G. Ho, L.S. Young, and R.P. Gale.(1979): Pneumococcal infections after human bone marrow transplantation. Ann.Int.Med. 91:835-841

Prevention of infections in patients with acute leukemia and granulocytopenia

D. van der Waaij, H.G. de Vries-Hospers

Laboratory for Medical Microbiology, University of Groningen, The Netherlands

INTRODUCTION
In the last years considerable progress has been made in the antimicrobial management of the immunocompromised host. A great number of antibiotics with broad-spectrum activity has been developed. The importance of prompty initiating emperic antibiotic therapy when the granulocytopenic patient becomes febrile is generalli recognized. This often expensive kind of parenteral treatment should be continued until resolution of granulocytopenia if no other precautions are taken to reduce the change for infection. Inherent to this approach is the change of development of drug resistance to valuable new antibiotics, particularly in Gram-negative bacilli. In case resistance develops, overgrowth of these resistant bacteria in the digestive tract may occur and possibly spread to other patients in the ward (Flynn DM et al, 1987).
On a haematologic oncologic ward, virtually all patients develop fever in the course of the second week of remission induction therapy. Therefore, many patients are often longterm antibiotic treatment with the same combinations of antibiotics. This unwanted situation could be avoided by using a somewhat different form of infection prevention in the immunocompromised patient. In this paper attention will be given to such a form of infection propylaxis directed against Gram-negative bacilli, yeastd and Staphylococcus aureus . For this kind of (selective) prophylactic treatment a long term antimicrobial treatment is required which is called Selective Decontamination of the Digestive tract (SDD). Because of the unique spectrum of the antimicrobial drugs that have been specially selected for SDD and because of the daily dosage of these drugs, the change of development of resistance among the Gram-negative bacilli which are the "target bacteria" of SDD, is minimal.
This new approach of infection prevention, which was first tested in

patients in late seventies, is <u>based on the fact that the indigenous - predominantly anaerobic - microflora of man, which comprisis of 99% of the total gastro-intestinal tract flora, has an important function in the defence against infection.</u> The great majority of the bacterial species which belong to the indigenous flora is pathogenic or of low pathogenicity and these strains control the population pattern in the digestive tract of pathogenic and potencially pathogenic bacteria as well as of yeasts. This mechanism which controls growth and persistance of potencially pathogenic (Gram-positive and Gram-negative) microorganism <u>is called Colonization resistance</u> (CR) (Van der Waaij D et al, 1971; Van der Waaij D et al, 1977; Berg RD, 1980). <u>Selective decontamination</u> consequently, is performed with antimicrobial drugs which are <u>selected for having no or minimal effect on the CR-associated part of the oral and intestinal microflora</u> (Berg RD, 1980). It concerns in general antimicrobial drugs which have a small spectrum of activity that excludes (Gram-positive) anaerobic intestinal bacteria.

SELECTIVE DECONTAMINATION OF THE DIGESTIVE TRACT (SDD)
For successful application of SDD insight is necessary in the underlying mechanism of this treatment. This implies a short explanation of why the indigenous flora is important and which kind of bacteria are involved. With this knowledge it will also be easier understood which antibiotics can safely be applied for systemic therapy for longer periods in neutropenic patients. Therefore, both aspects of "CR-safe" antimicrobial treatment - SDD and systemic theraphy - will be discussed separately in the following two paragraphs after a brief discussion of CR.

COLONIZATION RESISTANCE OF THE DIGESTIVE TRACT
Colonization resistance (CR) is the resistance which potentially pathogenic microorganisms encounter when they try to colonize one of the three tracts with open communication with the outside world (Van der Waaij D, 1971; Van der Waaij D, 1977). The presence of potencially pathogenic species of bacteria or yeasts and their number, may be of key importance for the development of infection in both the urinary and the respiratory tract (Berg RD, 1980; Tancrede CH et al, 1985). In the neutropenic patient most infections by potencially pathogenic microbes in these tracts find their sources in the digestive tract.

The CR of the digestive tract is the resultant of close cooperation between the host organism and its indigenous flora (Tancrede CH et al, 1985).

In healthy individuals, the intestinal flora consists largely of (many) anaerobic bacterial species, while in the oropharyngeal area in addition to (less) anaerobes streptococci colonize the mucosa predominantly as indigenous species (Van der Waaij D, 1982). For colonization of potentially pathogenic Gram-positive as well as Gram-negative bacteria, rather high oral doses of at least 10^6 are required. This figure is in bacteria-free animals or patients with an antibiotic decontaminated (sterilized) gut in the order of 10^5 lower (Buck AC et al, 1969; Cooke EM et al, 1972; Williams SH,1975). This means that extremely low oral contamination with about 100 bacteria can result in colonization of the oral cavity and the intestines. The same may occur in patients who are being systematically treated with broad-spectrum antibiotic combinations which are excreted with the saliva and into the intestines. Antibiotics may reach the contents of the alimentary canal either by incomplete absorbtion following oral administration, or during i.v.-treatment because of secretion with saliva, mucus or perhaps most important with the bile into the g.i.-tract. If along onnnnnne or all of these lines, the antibiotic concentrations in the digestive tract reaches the sensitivity level of the CR-associated (anaerobic) mucosa-associated flora, the degree decreases rapidly. The rapidity of this decrease depends on the level and the duration of a suppressive steady state level at mucosal level.

Antibiotic treatment and colonization resistance
In the foregoing paragraph, the importance of a normal indigenous flora in the immunocompromised patients has been discussed. When this was recognized in the early seventies, a series of animal experiments was set up to screen antibiotics for their effect on CR-constituting flora in mice (Thijm HA et al, 1979; Van der Waaij D et al, 1982; Van der Waaij D et al, 1982; Wiegersma N et al, 1982). In these experiments, groups of mice were treated with different daily doses of a particular antimicrobial drug for several weeks. During this treatment period, the concentration of opportunistic (potentially pathogenic) bacteria in the faeces was determined as well as other parameters of the CR were investigated at regular intervals. The results of these studies showed that antimicrobial drugs can roughly be subdivided in three major clesses (Wiegersma N et al, 1982):
1. Antibiotics which do affect the CR-associated microflora at any clinical dose level
2. Antibiotics which decrease the CR only when high clinically applicable doses are used
3. Antibiotics which do not decrease the CR, even not when applied in unusual high doses.
These differences appeared to be due to either complete absorbtion from the intestines (no antibiotic substance reaches then in most cases the RC-associated flora) or to the small spectrum which was limited to anti-Gram-negative activity (no activity to CR-associated predominantly Gram-positive flora; even not at high concentrations).
In paralel to traffic lights, the three groups of antimicrobials mentioned above could be refered to respectively "red" (CR-decreasing), "orange" (only

CR-affecting after high clinical doses) or "green" (no danger for the CR-flora).

In the screening experiments in mice, potentially pathogenic bacteria, that were susceptible to the antibiotic being screened, disappeared from the intestines (faeces) at a certain dose level. Only if the minimal CR-decreasing dose was fourfold or more (higher) than the "minimal pathogen aradicating dose", the drug was regarded "safe" for application in prophylactic treatment which soon became known as <u>selective decontamination of the digestive tract</u> (SDD) (Van der waaij D et al.,1974; Sleijfer DT et al.,1980; Dekker et al.,1981; Wade JC et al.,1983).If this dose level -the "minimal Gram-negative potential pathogen eradicating dose"- the CR-associated microflora appeared still unaffected, the drug was considered worth further studying for application for SDD, aiming infection prophylaxis in immunocompromised individuals.

In conclusion: SDD is accomplished in patients by oral treatment with "green" antimicrobial drugs in daily dosages which are sufficiently high to rapidly eliminate (within a week) the suceptible potentially pathogenic part of the flora.

Subsequent studies in man have learned that the intestinal (and oral) CR-constituting flora of mice and man respond similarly to antibiotics although differ significantly in composition (Dekker et al., 1981; Wade JC et al.,1983). Antibiotics which were labled "red" after screening in mice appear the same that in patients are generally associated with "bacterial overgrowth". "Green" antimicrobials on the other hand, have been found to be not toxic to the CR-constituting flora of man, even not when applied in doses high enough to eliminate the potential pathogenic bacteria that are susceptible to the drug(s) used. Examples of these antimicrobials are : co-trimoxazole, quinolones, polymyxins, polyenes and oral cephalosporins such as cephradine. Except for polymyxin and the polyenes however, these drugs have yet dose limitations; i.e. at extremely high daily doses they may affect the CR.

<u>Infection prevention by selective decontamination in granulocytopenic patients</u>

As soon as neutropenic patients are admitted to the ward or if their granulocyopenia is imminent because of remission induction chemotherapy, a comprehensive bacteriological inventory should be made. This includes cultures of throat, faeces, urine, vagina,prepucium and (pus from) lesions. These cultures are necessary to obtain inside in whether an infection is imminent or not. During SDD-treatment the surveillance cultures can be confined to those of the throat and faeces with a frequency of two or three times per week. When at inventory potential pathogens are cultured from one or more of the other sites, those cultures must be repeated until they have become negative as a result of SDD-tretment.

After bacteriological inventarisation, SDD can be started with drugs directed at three groups of microorganism:
1. Gram-negative (aerobic) rods; Enterobacteriaceae and Pseudomonaceae
2. Yeasts such as Candida and Torulopsis species
3. Staphylococcus eureus

ad 1. <u>Gram-negative bacilli</u> : These enteric bacteria can be eliminated by means of one or more of the antimicrobical drugs enlisted in Table 1.

Table 1. Drugs for selective decontamination, their target microorganism and the daily dose at which they should be applied.

Drugs for SDD	Target microorganisms	Daily dose for adults
Pipemidic acid	Enterobacteriaceae spp.	800 mg
Norfloxacin	" "	800 mg
Ciprofloxacin	" "	1000 mg
	some Pseudomonas	"
Co-trimoxazole	" "	6 regular tablets
	Staphylococcus aureus	"
Polymyxin B or E	most Enterobact. species	800 mg
	" Pseudomonas "	"
Cefradin	Staphylococcus aureus	6000 mg
Amphotericin B	Yeasts	2000 mg

A choice of SDD-drugs should be made on the basis of the susceptibility pattern of the potential pathogens found in the inventory of the flora. When there is no time to wait for the outcome of these cultures, treatment could be started with a combination of co-trimoxazolo and polimyxin B or E (colostin) (Rozenberg-Arska M et al.,1983).Another "best choice" could be one of the quinolones such as norfloxacin (Karp JE et al.,1988) or ciprofloxacin (Rozenberg-Arska M et al.,1985).
If the choice of antimicrobials for SDD is correct, faecal cultures are usually negative within a week of treatment.Obviously treatment must be continued to mantain the cultures negative until the increased risk of infection (leukopenia) is over.
In case the use of absorbable drugs is contra-indicated because of hypersensitivity for example, oral polymyxin with aztreonam is be considered (De Vries-Hospers HG et al.,1984). Negative faecal and oral cultures can be expected somewhat faster in with this treatment. However, on the other hand the systemic protection for a number of Gram-positive infections provided by absorbable drugs, fails in this case. In addition,although elimination of Gram-negative bacteria from the gut (faeces) is in general sufficiently rapidly achieved to prevent infections by the microbes targeted by the drugs employed from the gut, in the

oropharynx this may be more difficult. If Gram-negative bacilli are present in the oropharynx of the patient at onset and persist during SDD-treatment it is sometimes necessary to add absorbable SDD-drugs to the SDD-regimen chosen.. Expecially co-trimoxazole may be of help to clear the oropharyngeal area of aerobic
Gram-negative bacilli.

In case co-trimoxazole treatment is contra-indicated for completing SDD treatment in the oropharynx, local application of a sticky creme called "orabase" premixed with 2% of SDD-drugs is be considered. This sticky substance has a poor compliance and most patients are not prepared to applicate this creme on their gums three as they should for optimal effect. If necessary, one could start with the application of orabase during sleeping hours at night.

Possible infectious foci in the oropharyngeal area such as peridontitis or sinusitis must not be overlooked. If necessary, these sources for a generalized infection later during remission induction therapy should be disinfected and treated as a seperate entity (seperate to the general procedures discussed for the digestive tract).

ad 2. Yeasts :   In contrast to for the Gram-negative bacilli, the oropharynx is an important, site for colonization of yeasts. Without antimycotic treatment, more than 50% of the granulocytopenic patients usually become colonized by Candida or Torulopsis species. From the oropharyngeal area the digestive tract becomes easily infected down stream. This among else may result in positive faecal culture for these yeasts.

For selective suppression of colonization of yeasts in the digestive tract, either amphotericin B or nystatin can be used. Because of better sensitivity of yeasts for ampho-B we prefer ampho-B. To optimalize the drug activity in the oropharynx, this drug can best be given as a suspencion.

In spite of attempts to optimalize yeast suppression, cultures remain often positive, albeit due to low numbers of yeast cells. In case a patient is admitted heavily colonized, application of lozenges with ampho-B is to be considered for more rapid reduction of yeasts colonization. By sucking lozenges with ampho-B, this polyene antibiotic is gradually released and mixed with saliva in the course of one to two hours (De Vries-Hospers HG et al., 1982). The addition of lozenges is particularly advocated when the patient has mucosal lesions, "clinically suspected for Candida/Torulopsis infection". Also, if foreign bodies such as a nasogastric tube for hyperalimentation are present. Finally, a denture should be weared, except during the meals and visiting time.

ad 3. Staphylococcus aureus : This staphylococcal species (but not Staph. epidermidis) can also be selectively eliminated by antimicrobial treatment. By daily oral treatment with cefradin (an oral cephalsporin)

sensitive Staph. aureus normally disappears, generally in the course of on average three days from the oropharingeal-, nose- and faecal cultures. Treatment can generally be stopped after three weeks of treatment without recurrence of these staphylococci. Stopping of oral/systemic cefradin treatment could be considered even sooner if co-trimixazole is being used for suppression of Gram-negative bacilli. In our experience only about 10% of the patients require cefradine treatment because of positive surveillance cultures; the majority is negative at admission and remains so during SDD-treatment.
General : All drug used for selective suppression of Gram-negative bacilli and yeast should be given as long as the peripheral granulocyte count is below $0.5 \times 10^9/l$ of blood.

FOOD

Usually SDD-patients are not isolated and they can eat the normal non-sterile but carefully hygenically prepared hospital food. Food known to be often rather heavily contaminated like raw meat, salads etc should be avoided; (family) visitors should not bring any food from outside the hospital.
Patients with insufficient oral intake can be fed parenterally or be feeding via a nasogastric tube. In case of enteral hyperalimentation we recommend the use of sterile food suspencion because these food suspencion get easily contaminated and are very rich media for bacterial growth; often of potentially pathogenic bacteria.

ADVERSE EFFECT

Adverse effects due to SDD-treatment such as nausea, skin rash may occur. Allergic reactions are especially seen in patients who are treated with co-trimoxazole; nausea occurs occasinally because of treatment with ampho-B suspencion. Prolonged duration of granulocytopenia ascribed to the use of co-trimoxazole has been reported by two investigators (Dekker et al., 1981; Wade JC et al., 1983).

SYSTEMIC TREATMENT DURING SDD

Succesfully selectively decontaminated patients should be free of potentially pathogenic Gram-negative bacilli and Sthaph. aureus and should be colonized by only a minimal number of yeasts. They should not develop infections by these organisms. Gram-positive infections by oral streptococci and Staph. epidermidis (i.e. other than Staph. aureus) however, still occur. Therefore when patients develop fever, careful consideration of the various possible reasons for fever is necessary. When allergic reaction due to drugs or transfusions can be excluded as a reason, prompt institution of a combination of cidal antibiotics is indicated while SDD-treatment obviously must be continued meanwhile in order to mantein

SDD successful. The choice of antibiotics for systemic therapy should be guided by the most recent findings in the surveillance cultures if they have been positive in the recent past (last two weeks).
If possible, for therapy, preference should be given to broad -spectrum antibiotics which do not or minimally affect the CR-associated microflora (Nord CE et al., 1984). In the selection of antibiotics for emperic therapy, the sensitivity pattern of streptococci and Staph. epidermidis should be taken into account.
General : Before institution of intravenous antibiotic therapy a sufficient number of blood samples should be taken for culturing. In case (one of) these cultures is positive, treatment can be adjusted to the outcome of the sensitivity testing of the isolate.

DEVELOPMENT OF RESISTANCE DURING SDD
During the many years of SDD-treatment since 1976 in our hospital, development of resistance in Gram-negative bacilli was not seen during treatment. It was however, been observed occasionally in the first week of treatment in the initial period (till 1980) when nalidixic acid was applied (as a single drug) for SDD-treatment (De Vries-Hospers HG et al., 1981).
An epidemiological positive side effect of SDD is that in a haematological ward in which exclusively granulocytopenic are being treated, cross-infection with Gram-negative bacilli does not occur when for SDD-treatment of all patients in the ward SDD-drug(s) are used which are effective to the Gram-negatives of each newly arriving patient ; otherwise new patients should be manteined isolated until the outcome of their admission cultures is known and appears free of (multi-)resistant Gram-negatives.

REFERENCES

Berg RD, (1980) Inhibition of translocation from the gastrointestinal tract by normal cecal flora in gnotobiotic and antibiotic decontaminated mice Inf. Immun. 29, 1073-1081

Buck AC,Cooke EM (1969) The fate of ingested Pseudomonas Aeruginosa in normal persons J. Med. Microbiol. 2, 521-525

Cooke EM,Hettiaratchy GT,Buck AC (1972) Fate of ingested Escherichia coli in normal persons J. Med. Microbiol. 5, 361-369

Dekker, Rozenberg-Arska M,Sixma JJ,Erhoef J (1981) Prevenction of infection by trimethoprim-sulfamethoxazole plus amphotericin B in patients with acute nonlymphocytic leukemia N. Engl. J. Med. 95, 555-559

De Vries-Hospers HG, Slijefer DT, Mulder NH, Van der Waaij D, Nieweg HO, Van Saene HKF (1981) Bacteriological aspects of the digestive tract as a method of infection prevention in granulocytopenic patients Antimicrob. Ag. Chemother 19, 813-820

De Vries-Hospers HG, Mulder NH, Sleijfer DT, Van Saene HKF (1982) The effect of amphotericin B lozenges on the presence and number of Candida cells in the oropharynx of neutropenic leukemia patients Infection 10, 71-85

De Vries-Hospers HG, Welling GW, Swabb EA, Van der Waaij D (1984) Selective decontamination of the digestive tract with aztreonam : a study in 10 healthy volunteers J. Inf. Dis. 150, 636-641

Flynn DM, Weinstein CN, Gaston MA, Kabins SA (1987) Patients' endogenous flora as the source of "nosocomial" Enterobacter in cardiac surgery J Inf Dis 156, 363-368

Karp JE, Dick JD, Merz WG (1988) Systemic infection and colonization with and without prophylactic norfloxacin use over time in granulocytopenic, acute leukemia patients Eur. J. Cancer Clin. Oncol. 24 suppl., 1 : 5-13

Nord CE, Kager L, Heimdahl A. (1984) Impact of antimicrobial agents on the gastrointestinal microflora and the risk of infections Am. J. Med. 76, 99-106

Rozenberg-Arska M, Dekker AW, Verhoef J (1983) Colistin and trimethoprim-sulfamethoxazole for prevention of infection in patients with acute nonlymphocyttic leukemia. Decrease in the emergence of resistant bacteria Infection 11, 167-169

Rozenberg-Arska M, Dekker AW, Verhoef J (1985) Ciprofloxacin for selective decontamination of the alimentary tract in patients with acute leukemia during remission induction treatment; the effect of faecal flora J. Inf. Dis 152, 104-107

Sleijfer DT, Mulder NH, De Vries-Hosper HG et al. (1980) Infection prevenction in granulocytopenic patients by selective decontamination of the digestive tract Eur. J. Cancer 16, 859-869

Tancrede CH, Andremont AO (1985) Bacterial translocation and Gram-negative bacteriemia in patients with hematological malignancies J. Inf. Dis. 152, 99-103

Thijm HA,Van der Waaij D (1979) The effect of three frequently applied antibiotics on the colonization resistance of the digestive tract in mice J. Hyg. 82, 397-404

Van der Waaij D,Berghuis-de Vries JM,Lekerkerk-van der Wees JEC (1971) Colonization resistance of the digestive tract in conventional and antibiotic treated mice J. Hyg. 60, 405-411

Van der Waaij D,Berghuis-de Vries JM (1974) Selective elimination of Enterobacteriaceae species from the digestive tract in mice and monkey J. Hyg. 72, 205-211

Van der Waaij D,Vossen JM,Korthals Altes C,Hartgrink C (1977) Reconventionalization following antibiotic decontamination in man and animal Am. J. Nutr. 30, 1887-1895

Van der Waaij D (1979) In New criteria for antimicrobial therapy : maintenance of colonization resistance., eds. Van der WaaijD,Verhoef J, pp. 271-280. Amsterdam,Oxford : Excepta Medica

Van der Waaij D (1982) In Action of antibiotic in patients , ed. Sabath LD,pp 104-118. Bern,Stuttgart, Vienna : Hans Huber Publisher

Van der Waaij D. In Medical Microbiology, eds Easmon CSF,Jeljaszewicz J. pp. 227-237. London : Academic Press Inc.

Van der Waaij D,Aberson, Thijm HA,Welling GW (1982) The screening of four aminoglycosides in the selective decontamination of the digestive tract in mice Infection 10, 35-40

Van der Waaij D,Hofstra G,Wiegersma N (1982) Effect of betalactam antibiotics on the resistance of the digestive tract to colonization J. Inf. Dis. 146, 417-422

Wade JC,De Jongh CA,Newman KA,Crowley J,Wiernick PH,Schimpff SC (1983) Selective antimicrobial modulation as prophylaxis against infection during granulocytopenia : trimethoprim-sulfamethoxazole vs nalidixic acid J. Inf. Dis. 147, 624-634

Wiegersma N,Jansen,Van der Waaij D (1982) J. Hyg. 88, 221-230

Williams Smith H. (1975) Survival of orally administred E. Coli in the alimentary tract of man Nature 225, 500-502

Infections in bone marrow transplantation: a comparison between allogeneic and autologous graft

S. Tura, P. Ricci, G. Bandini, E. Calori, L. Albertazzi, G. Rosti, F. Verlicchi, A.M. Foralosso, G. Poletti

Istituto di Ematologia "L. e A. Seragnoli», Bologna, Italy

INTRODUCTION

Infections constitute, directly or indirectly, the main cause of bone marrow transplantation-associated morbidity and mortality. Risk factors for infections vary with time in the post transplant period and also influence different etiologic agents. This topic has been reviewed extensively (Meyers, 1986; Watson, 1983, Young, 1984; Winston, 1984) and a brief summary is given here.
Early post-BMT infections before bone marrow engraftment (until day 20). Risk factors are epidemiologic milieu of the patient and of the transplant unit, profound neutropenia, indwelling central venous catheters and short term extra-hematologic toxicity of pretransplant conditioning. The most common proved infection is bacteriemia; rarer, but much more severe, is Candida septicemia. The once very frequent complication of oropharingeal HSV reactivation is now of less clinical relevance following the widespread use of intravenous acyclovir. Approaches to the prevention of infections are a protected enviroment, total or selective intestinal decontamination with oral antibiotics, sterile or low-bacterial-content diet, i.v. acyclovir and high dose immunoglobulins. Treatment of infections consists of three subsequent steps: 1) immediate empirical wide spectrum i.v. antibiotic therapy in febrile patients; 2) adjustment of therapy in accordance with colture results; 3) empirical i.v. amphotericin and/or granulocyte transfusions in the event of persistance of fever.
Early post-BMT infections after engraftment (from day 20 to 100). Risk factors are cellular and humoral immunodeficiency, medium term extra-hematologic toxicity of the conditioning regime, occurrence of acute GVHD and its treatment. The major infections are viral (CMV, adenovirus and VZV), non bacterial interstitial pneumonia (CMV, Pneumocystis and idiopathic), bacterial, candidal and aspergillar infections. Prevention begins in the first phase

of transplant with the choice of fractionated Total Body Irradiation or very low dose rates (Weiner, 1986)and use of CMV antibody negative blood donors (Bowden, 1986). Prevention continues, expecially in patients with acute GVHD, with passive immunophrophylaxis, acyclovir or D.H.P.G. (Shepp, 1985) and cotrimoxazole. Therapy is based on the etiolologic assessment of the infection; D.H.P.G.(CMV), acyclovir (VZV), cotrimoxazole (Pneumocystis), colture based antibiotics (bacterial and fungal infections).

Late post-BMT infections (after day 100).

Risk factors are evolving of immune reconstitution, chronic GVHD and its treatment. Common infections are localized VZ and upper respiratory tract infections from encapsulated bacteria. Prevention is limited to patients with chronic GVHD and consists of cotrimoxazole administration per os and regular i.v. immunoglobulins.

Since 1982 BMT was given to 116 adult patients with haematologic malignancies: they were nursed under identical conditions and were given the same nutritional, transfusional and general support. In 44 patients the graft was autologous, using cryopreserved marrow; in 72 cases the graft was from HLA identical siblings. We have compared the incidence of infections in the two groups during the hospitalization period of transplant and subsequently from discharge to day 100, from day 101 to one year and beyond this point. The aim of the study is the definition of risk factors and the assessment of their importance in causing infections.

PATIENTS AND METHODS

The main characteristics of the two groups of patients undergoing allogeneic (BMT) and autologous bone marrow transplantation (ABMT) are shown in table 1.

During the transplant procedure the patients stayed in the same ward and received the same nutritional, transfusional and general support. They were isolated in single protected rooms and were given low-bacterial diet and oral antibiotics (Cotrimoxazole or NEOCO regime plus Nystatin). Intravenous acycloguanosine was used for the prophylaxis or treatment of the early oropharingeal infections. Immunoprophylaxis with high dose i.v. immunoglobulins was performed irregularly in a small number of patients in both groups. After discharge all patients continued or Nystatin or oral Amphotericin B for at least 3 months. Patients with GVHD receved chronic cotrimoxale.

Table 1: Main characteristics of the two groups of patients undergoing allogeneic (BMT) and autologous bone marrow transplantation (ABMT).

	ABMT	BMT
Patients	44	72
Age (median & range)	30 (15-51)	32 (13-50)
Sex (M / F)	25/19	42/30
Diagnosis:		
CML	0	34
ANLL	10	22
NHL	30	1
MYELOMA	1	11
ALL	1	4
HL	2	0

Table 2 shows the conditioning regimens used in the two groups of patients.

Table 2: Conditioning regime in the two groups of patients.

	ABMT	BMT
TBI + CTX	17	21
TBI + CTX + other drugs	2	49
BAVC (1)	21	0
CTX + BUSULFAN	4	2

(1) BAVC regime consists of BCNU 200 mg/m^2 on day -4, ARA-C 150 mg/m^2 q 12 hrs, VP-16 150 mg/m^2 q 12 hrs and CTX 45 mg/kg q 24 hrs from day -5 to day -2.

Patients undergoing BMT were fully HLA- identical, MLR unreactive with their sibling donors. GVHD prophylaxis was attempted with Cyclosporin-A (CSA) in 44 patients, with T-depletion in 17 and with CSA & MTX in 11 patients.

Table 3 shows the dose of infused marrow, speed of haematologic recovery, duration of hospitalization, duration of severe neutropenia, duration of i.v. antibiotic therapy, incidence of documented bacterial and fungal infections and transplanted related mortality, in the two groups of patients.

Table 3: Dose of infused marrow, hematological reconstitution and main clinical events from day 0 to discharge.

	ABMT	BMT	P
Patients	44	72	
Marrow cells infused/kg x10^8	2,1±0,7	3,1±1,3	<0,001
GM-CFU infused/kg x 10^4	8,0±6,8	35,5±35,0	<0,001
Days to 500 PMNs	19±8	16±4	NS
Days to 500 lymphocytes	16±8	26±14	<0,001
Days to 50000 platelets	15±4	15±4	NS
Days in hospital post-BMT:			
all patients	24±11	32±11	=0,02
surviving patients	26±10	30±9	=0,018
Days with < 100 PMNs	8±4	4±4	<0,001
Days with fever (>38°C)	7±7	7±7	NS
Days with i.v. antibiotics	16±11	16±11	NS
Documented infections (1)	26	28	=0,054
Interstitial pneumonia (I.P.)	0	1(2)	NS
Transplant related deaths	1	10	=0,08

(1) bacterial or fungal sepsis and bacterial pneumonia
(2) I.P. from CMV and Pneumocistis Carinii in the same patient

The peripheral blood reconstitution was identical in the two groups despite the high differences in the doses of infused marrow and the freezing procedure performed in the autologous group. The marked difference in the lymphocyte recovery was clearly caused by GVHD prevention, GVHD and its therapy (see Table 3).

Table 4 shows the correlations between fever and neutropenia and documented infections and neutropenia (PMNs 500).

Table 4: Incidence of fever and correlation between fever and neutropenia and documented infections and neutropenia.

	ABMT	BMT	P
Patients	44	72	
Days with fever (>38°C)	298	476	NS
Days with fever in neutropenic period (<500PMNs)	260 (87%)	319 (67%)	0,001
Documented infections	26	28	=0,054
Documented infections in neutropenic period (<500PMNs)	25 (94%)	23 (82%)	NS

Days with fever and with i.v. antibiotics were identical in the two groups. The incidence of both bacterial and fungal infections was higher in the autologous group and this finding correlated with the number of days with < 100 PMNs.
The occurrence of documented infections, however did not influence the duration of hospital stay or affect the transplant related mortality during this period of time (see Table 3).
Systemic Candidiasis was the cause of death at day +16 in one patient only (Bandini, 1986). In the other instances of transplant related deaths bacterial or fungal infections were associated with failure to take or rejections (1 patient with ABMT and 2 with BMT) or complicated acute GVHD (aGVHD) of grade III/IV (2 patients).
The majority of documented infections in both groups occurred during neutropenia (< 500 PMN) however, the incidence of fever outside neutropenia was significantly higher in BMT patients and this finding was probably due to aGVHD or to an infectious cause that we could not assess (see Table 4).
Staphylococci, Pseudomonas and Candida accounted for most of the documented infections of this period. Viral infections were not a major problem in this early post-transplant period, being represented in most istances by the isolation of H.S.V. from the pharingeal "lavage" or tipical mucosal or cutaneous lesions. Only in two cases, where delayed acyclovir treatment was employed, did a severe oropharingeal mucositis develop. One patient with grade III skin aGVHD died of a combined CMV/Pneumocystis carinii interstitial pneumonia. (Table 5 and 6)
Table 5 and 6 show the incidence of documented bacterial and viral infections and their causative agents, respectively.

Table 5: Documented infections in the two groups.

	ABMT	BMT	P
Patients	44	72	
Bacterial sepsis	22	24	NS
Bacterial pneumonia	1	2	NS
Fungal sepsis	3	2	NS
Localized fungal infections	3	7	NS
Viral infections	12	21	NS

Table 6: Bacterial and fungal organism and viruses isolated in the two groups.

	ABMT	BMT
Staphylococcus epidermidis	8	10
Pseudomonas spp.	8	7
Others Gram +	4	6
Others Gram -	3	5
Candida albicans	6	9
Herpes Simplex	12	20
Herpes Zoster	0	1
Cytomegalovirus	0	1

Post transplant infections from discharge to day 100.

For the purpose of this analysis we have considered patients with a follow-up > 2 months or those who died of infection within two months of transplant. In Table 7 the infections of this period in the two groups of patients are compared.

Table 7: Infectious complications from discharge to day 100.

	ABMT	BMT	P
Patients	40	62	
Bacterial sepsis	2	5	NS
Bacterial pneumonia	1	2	NS
Fungal infections	0	2 (1)	NS
Pneumonia of U.O.	1	2	NS
"Idiopathic" I.P.	2	2	NS
I.P. from CMV	0	5	NS
VZV infection	2	4	NS
TOTAL	8	22	NS
Transplant related deaths	2 (2)	7(3)	NS

(1) Oral esophageal candidiasis.
(2) Sepsis (1 pt) and total body failure (1 pt)
(3) I.P. from CMV (5 pt), cerebral hemorrage (1 pt), GVHD and infection (1 pt).

During this period infections did not represent a significant problem for patients in the ABMT group. Only one patient died of infection (bacterial sepsis). In 3 cases a clinico-radiological picture of mild interstitial pneumonia developed, and responded promptly to low-dose steroid therapy. Of the BMT patients, mainly those with aGVHD had bacterial and/or fungal infections and several episodes of fever of undetermined origin. Those complications were generally controlled easily with antibiotics, steroids, and antifungal agents per os. Interstitial pneumonia developed in 7 patients of the allogeneic group.

The diagnostic work-up included bronchoscopy with coltural studies, cytologic examination of broncho-alveolar lavage. and transbronchial biopsy. In 5 cases CMV was diagnosed and all pts died with respiratory failure despite aggressive treatment including D.H.P.G. and iperimmune specific IgG.

Two cases of "idiopathic" I.P. responded to steroid, 6-7 with I.P. also had cutaneous grade II or III GVHD.

Tipical VZV infections developed in 8 patients (2 with ABMT and 6 with BMT) and were always well controlled by i.v. acyclovir. In both groups a reactivation of oropharingeal H.S. was often observed but the incidence was much higher in the recipients of BMT who had GVHD.

Late post-transplant infections.

We have analysed two periods from day 101 to 1 year and after 1 year. Patients included in the first period were those with a survival of at least 6 months or patients with a follow-up 6 months but who had infection after day 101.

In the second period we have included all patients with a follow-up 1 year. Infections of this two period are shown in Table 8. They represented a minor problem in the ABMT group, where 5 VZV localized infections occurred. Patients who received BMT, on the contrary, continued with very frequent infections, often severe and in same instances constituting the main cause of death.

Polmonary complications of different nature and etiology occurred in 35 cases and were the cause of death in 6 patients. Interstitial pneumonias represented an important problem till the 6th month post-BMT, then became very rare. In 7 cases bronchoscopy + B.A.L. and biopsy could not allow to make a diagnosis. In 6 out of 7 pts therapy with steroids determined a clinical and radiological remission. In the seventh patient, however, disease progressed and he died of respiratory failure.

Table 8: Late post-transplant infections.

	from day 101 to 1 year			After 1 year		
	ABMT	BMT	P	ABMT	BMT	P
Patients	37	55		31	32	
Bacterial sepsis	2(1)	2	NS	0	2	NS
Bacterial pneumonia	0	5	NS	0	1	NS
Fungal infections	1	1	NS	0	0	NS
Fungal pneumonia	0	1	NS	0	0	NS
Pulmonary tubercolosis	0	1	NS	0	0	NS
Pneumonia of U.O.	1	5	NS	0	10	=0,005
"Idiopatic" I.P.	0	7	=0.06	0	1	NS
I.P. from CMV	0	3	NS	0	0	NS
I.P. from P.C.	0	1	NS	0	0	NS
VZV infection	4	14	NS	1	7	=0,065
HIV infection	0	0	NS	0	1(3)	NS
TOTAL	8	40	0,001	1	22	<0,001
Transplant related deaths	0	7(2)	=0,04	0	1(4)	NS

(1) in relapse (1 pt.), very slow p.b. reconstitution (1 pt.).
(2) fungal pneumonia (1 pt.), pulmonary tbc (1 pt.), Idiopathic I.P. (1 pt.), I.P. from CMV (2 pts.), I.P. from PC (1 pt.).
(3) from marrow donor.
(4) chronic GVHD.

Two of the three patients with CMV/I.P. died. TheTwo of the three had a clinical response with steroids and the pulmonary picture progressed to localized fibrosis. This I.P. was characterized by the late onset (7 months after BMT vs. less than 4 mos. for all the others). All the patients who developed idiopathic or CMV I.P. had aGVHD (mostly grade II or III of the skin) or had mild chronic GVHD. Pneumonias of undetermined origin developed very often, but never caused the patient's death and responded to wide spectrum antibiotics.
Twenty-one patients had localized or generalized VZV infection, in all cases controlled by acyclovir.

CONCLUSIONS

The comparison of infectious complications of two groups of patients undergoing BMT or ABMT at the same transplant unit allows to make some observations.
1) In the early post-transplant period infections were numerous and happened as frequently with ABMT as with BMT. The most important risk factor was represented by agranulocytosis, coupled with the toxicity of the conditioning regime on the mucosal barriers and the use of long term undwelling central venous catheters. The impact of aGVHD, in this period, was a significantly longer period of febrile days outside the neutropenic period. Infections were rarely the primary cause of death. More often transplant related deaths were due to the association of infection with aGVHD, failure to take or rejection.
2) After hematologic reconstitution, infections had a low incidence in the ABMT group. On the contrary, infections were very commmon in the BMT group and were the main cause of transplanted related deaths. It appears that the short and medium term extra-haematologic toxicity of the conditioning regimen is a minor risk factor.
Conversely, a determing risk factor is the type of immunologic reconstitution, whic is negatively influenced by GVHD prevention, GVHD itself and its therapy.

BIBLIOGRAFY

Bandini G., Ricci P, Guardigli C. et al. (1986): Unexpected presentation of deep candidiasis in a recipient of a mismatched bone marrow transplant. Acta Haematol. 75, 116.
Bowden R.A., Sayers M., Flournoy N. et al.(1986):Cytomegalovirus immunoglobulin and seronegative blood products to prevent primary cytomegalovirus infection after marror transplantation. New Engl. J.Med. 314, 1006.
Young, L.S. (1984): An overview of infection in bone marrow transplant recipients. Clin.in Haematology Oct.13 (3), 661-678.
Meyers, J.D (1986):Infections in bone marrow recipients.Am.J.Med.,July 81 1-A, 27-38.
Shepp D.H., Dandliker P.S., De Mirand P. et al. (1985): Activity of 9- (2-hydroxy-1-(hydroxymethy)

ethoxy-methilguanine in the treatment of cytomegalovirus pneumonia. Ann.Inter.Med. 103, 368-73.

Watson, J.G (1983): Problems of infections after bone marrow transplantation. J.Clin.Patol. 36, 683-692.

Weiner R.S., Bortin M.M., Gale R.P. et al.(1986): Interstitial pneumonities after bone marrow transplantation: assessment of risk factors. Ann. Int.Med. 104, 168-175.

Winston, D.J., Winston G.H., Champlin R.C., Gale R.P. (1984): Infectiuos complications of bone marrow transplantation. Exp.Haematol. 12, 205-215.

Infectious complications in acute myeloid leukemia in complete remission treated with high dose chemotherapy and autologous bone marrow transplantation

D. Caldera, E.P. Alessandrino, P. Bernasconi, M. Boni, E. Orlandi, G. Pagnucco, C. Castagnola, C. Bernasconi

Divisione di Ematologia, Policlinico S. Matteo IRCCS, Pavia, Italy

SUMMARY

Infectious complication is one of the major barrier to the success of ABMT. We evaluated the incidence of infections in 17 patients affected with Acute Myeloid Leukemia in Complete Remission, submitted to ABMT. Fever occurred in the 87 per cent of the patients: the incidence of microbiologically documented infections was 50 per cent, with a great prevalence of Gram+ infections (70 per cent). The adequate antibiotic therapy and the marrow recovery induced a full resolution of infections. We didn't notice any cases of infection related death.

KEYWORDS

Autologous Bone Marrow Transplantation, infectious complications.

INTRODUCTION

There is some evidence that Autologous Bone Marrow Transplantation (ABMT) in patients affected with Acute Myeloid Leukemia in Complete Remission (CR), prolongs remission duration and survival. The conditioning regimen used to eradicate residual disease induces a transient immunodeficiency, which predisposes to infectious complications. Main risk factors predisposing to infections are the loss of mucosal integrity, the transient aplasia, the profound impairment of most immune functions.
Seventeen patients with Acute Myeloid Leukemia in CR, submitted, for consolidation of remission, to high dose chemotherapy and Autologous Bone Marrow Transplantation, have been evaluated to assess the incidence of infectious complications related to the procedure.

PATIENTS AND METHODS

Between August 1985 and May 1988, seventeen patients affected with AML referred to Haematology Division of Pavia, were submitted, for consolidation of the remission, to high dose chemotherapy and Autologous Bone Marrow Transplantation: the patients mean age was 38 (21-49) years; 10 out of them were females and 7 males; at the time of bone marrow collection 9 patients were in first CR, 7 in second CR, 1 in third CR. For all the patients the conditioning regimen consisted of: BCNU mg 800/mq/24h i.v. on day -5, Citarabine mg 300/mq/24h i.v. continous infusion plus Etoposide mg 300/mq/24h i.v. on days -4-3-2. Prophylaxis of endogenous infections was appronted by: muco-cutaneous decontamination with antiseptic solution, gut selective decontamination with Cotrimoxazole g 1x2/die, antifungal therapy with Amphotericin B per os g1x2/die, surveillance coltures, additional viral bacterial and fungal coltures as required. The prophylaxis of exogenously acquired infections consisted of: protected environment, reverse barrier nursing, diet low in microbial content. The febrile episodes were treated with an empirical first line association of Cefotaxime mg 50/Kg/die plus Gentamicin mg 3-5/kg/die; as second line association we used Amikacin mg 15/Kg/die plus Piperacillin mg 150/Kg/die.

RESULTS

Only 16 of 17 patients on study were evaluable for infection risk: one patient, 38 year male, died in fourth day post-ABMT for acute renal failure. The mean inpatient stay was 33 (21-58) days, the mean duration of aplasia was 11 (9-20) days; fever occurred in 14 patients, mean duration of ever was 6 (1-18) days and the mean duration of antibiotic-therapy was 10 (1-23) days. The data related to the febrile episodes are reported in Table 1.

Table 1 - Febrile Episodes and Infectious Complications

- Evaluable patients	16
- Patients with febrile episodes	14 (87%)
- Conditioning regimen related fever	2 (14%)
- FUO	5 (35%)
- Documented infections: total	7 (50%)
sepsis	3
localized infections	4
- Infection related deaths	0

In seven cases we made a diagnosis of microbiologically documented infection: 1 Streptococcus D sepsis, 2 Staphylococcus Aureus sepsis, 3 catheter infections by Pseudomonas Aeruginosa, Staphylococcus Aureus, Staphylococcus coag-neg., 1 gum abscess by Pseudomonas spp.
We obtained a full resolution of infections in all cases. Clinical patients improvment occurred with marrow recovery. In addition we observed 1 case of B Hepatitis at day +35 and 1 cases of nonA-nonB Hepatitis at day +58.

DISCUSSION

In our experience all the febrile episodes occurred in patients with a neutrophil count less than 1×10^9 /L, and a full resolution was observed at the time of the marrow recovery. These data confirm that a temporal relationship exists between the onset of neutropenia and infections, and between the risk of infectious complications and the absolute neutrophil count (Bodey, 1966). In neutropenic patients infections are most commonly due to the Gram- organisms, but the postgrafting prophylaxis for the endogenously acquired infections and the use of central line catheters have led to the increase in the incidence of Gram+ infections. In our study this figure has been noticed in 5 out of 7 cases with microbiologically documented infection (71 per cent).
Some authors underlined that the early institution of empirical broad-spectrum antibiotic therapy in febrile neutropenic patients induces an overall reduction in mortality, from 50 per cent to 5 per cent (Schimpff, 1979). According to these data in our Division we started broad-spectrum antibiotic therapy whenever fever occurred for more than 4 hours: the first line empiric antibiotic association was able to control the 50 per cent of febrile episodes; the second line therapy resulted well fitted in the 43 per cent. In one patient we utilized Vancomycin, according to coltural data showing the presence of Staphylococcus coag-neg. (catheter infection). In the management of neutropenic patient with infection an intriguing point is how long to continue antibiotic therapy after the disappearance of the fever: in our cases we stoped the antibiotic therapy only when the neutrophil count returned to 1×10^9 /L. As far as this point is concerned, Pizzo (1979) reported that a short course of antibiotic therapy may induce a recrudesence of infection. Klastersky (1983) comparing patients who had a short course antibiotic therapy with patients who continued the therapy until the neutrophil level excedeed 0.5×10^9/L, didn't find significative difference in incidence of mortality.
In our study all the febrile episodes occurred during the postgrafting neutropenia; two patients developed viral hepatitis, at day +35 and +58 respectively. This event may be related to immunodeficiency and to supportive transfusional therapy. Patients submitted to bone marrow transplant, develop a transient immunodeficiency predisposing to late viral infections. A full reconstitution of the immunity may be achieved within one to two years from the transplant (Lum, 1987): during this period patients

need accurate infectivological surveillance.

CONCLUSION

Despite the use of prophylactic measures (isolation, reverse barrier nursing, gut and skin decontamination) infectious complications constitute the major problem in postgrafting: in our study fever occurred in 87 per cent of patients; 7 cases (43 per cent) developed a microbiological documented infection. Areas in which there is urgent need for developments include the rapid diagnosis of bacterial, viral and fungal infections, the use of new powerfull antibiotics for empirical therapy, the use of measures shortening the period of severe aplasia.

REFERENCES

Bodey G.P., Buckley M., Sathe V.S. et al (1966): Quantitative relationship between circulating leukocytes and infection in patients with acute leukemia. Ann. Int. Med. 64, 328-344.

Klastersky J. (1983): A cooperative trial of empiric treatment in febrile neutropenic patients. The third EORTC Trial International Chemotherapy Congress. Abstracts 71, 33-35.

Lum L.G. (1987): The kinetics of immune reconstitution after human marrow transplantation. Blood 69, 2, 369-380.

Pizzo P.A. Robichaud S.K., Gill F.A., Witelsky F.G., Levinse A.S., Deisseroth A.B. et al. (1979): Duration of empiric antibiotic therapy in granulocytopenic patients with cancer. Am. J. Med. 67, 194-200.

Schimpff S.C., Aisner J., Wiernik P.M. (1979): Infection in acute non-lymphocytic leukemia: the alimentary canal as a major source of pathogens. In: Van der Vaaj D., Verhoen J. (eds). New criteria for antimicrobial therapy. Amsterdam, Excerpta Medica, pp 12-29.

Infections and haemorrhage in acute leukaemia, T. Barbui, A. Falanga, B. Minetti, S. Gorini, G. Tognoni and M.D. Donati, eds. John Libbey Eurotext, Paris © 1989, pp. 141-145

Infection in neutropenic patients. Epidemiology at local institutions : preliminary results of an italian collaborative study

GISIN (Gruppo Italiano per lo Studio delle Infezioni nel Neutropenico) :
A. Del Favero[2], G. Bucaneve[2], P. Martino[1], F. Menichetti[3], B. Minetti[4], C. Viscoli[5], G. Todeschini[6], M. Rossi[7], G. Rocchi[8], G. Papa[8], U. Marinoni[9], S. Pauluzzi[3], P. Serra[10], A. Terragna[5]

[1] *Universita' di Roma, Cattedra di Ematologia,* [2] *Universita' di Perugia, Clinica Medica,* [1 e 3] *Universita' di Perugia, Istituto di Malattie Infettive,* [4] *Divisione di Ematologia Ospedale di Bergamo,* [5] *Universita' di Genova, I Clinica di Malattie Infettive, Istituto G. Gaslini,* [6] *Universita' di Verona, Cattedra di Ematologia, Policlinico Borgo Roma,* [7] *Clinica Pediatrica, Ente Ospedaliero di Monza,* [8] *II Universita' di Roma, Cattedra di Malattie Infettive e Cattedra di Ematologia,* [9] *ULSS 8 Regione Lombardia, Ospedale Busto Arsizio,* [10] *Istituto G. Galliera, Genova, Italy*

ABSTRACT
Poiche' i dati relativi alla epidemiologia delle infezioni nei pazienti neoplastici neutropenici risultano scarsi nel nostro paese, il G.I.S.I.N., un gruppo costituito da 35 istituzioni, ad orientamento prevalentemente ematologico ed infettivologico, distribuite in 16 citta', ha iniziato uno studio prospettico sulle infezioni in questi pazienti. Sono presentati i dati relativi ai primi 269 episodi febbrili raccolti in 9 centri.

KEY WORDS : Epidemiology, Infections, Neutropenic patients

INTRODUCTION
Infections remains a major complication and the leading cause of deaths in patients with malignant diseases (Inagaki 1974) and neutropenia is the most important predisposing factor in these patients. A prevalence of gram-negative infections in neutropenic patients has been observed in many centres and in several clinical trials, but the isolation of gram-positive pathogens from patients with cancer has increased notably over the past few years (Pizzo 1978).
As the knowledge on epidemiology of infections in neutropenic patients in our country is at best scanty, the G.I.S.I.N., an italian cooperative group including 35 institutions, mainly hematological and of infectious diseases located in 16 town, was set up in May 1987, and a prospective study , aimed at evaluating the epidemiology of infections occurring in febrile neutropenic patients admitted at the partecipating centres, was started in January 1988.

PATIENTS AND METHODS
Consecutive febrile episodes occurring in neutropenic cancer patients admitted at the partecipating institutions were studied. Patients were elegible if they had an absolute granulocyte count below 1000/mmc and an axillary temperature of 38° C or more in absence of obvious noninfective causes of fever. For each febrile episode the data on patient characteristics, classification of infection, antibiotic therapy and outcome were recorded using a

standardized computerized report form including more than 90 items. Febrile episodes were classified according to the EORTC definitions (EORTC, 1987). All bacterial isolates were identified by standard techniques and antimicrobial susceptibility was tested. Any modification of the initial antibiotic therapy was recorded. An overall evaluation was made at the end of the febrile episode. Any deaths observed during the febrile episode was charged in overall mortality; deaths were considered to be due to infection according to investigator's judgment. The data were stored and elaborated using SAS computing system.

RESULTS and DISCUSSIONS

Over a 5 month period 279 febrile episodes were studied at nine institutions (85% of cases were recorded by 4 centres), and 269 (232 patients) were considered evaluable for the analysis.
Patient characteristics are illustrated in Table 1. It should be noted that the majority of patients (58%) was affected by acute leukemia and that 50% of febrile episodes occurred in profoundly neutropenic (< 100/mmc) patients. Noteworthy is the fact that 65 % of patients received oral antimicrobial prophylaxis (mainly quinolones or co-trimoxazole) and 39% had a central venous catheter in place at the beginning of febrile episode. The 269 febrile episodes were classified as follow : microbiologically documented infection (38%) (with bacteremia 33.5%), clinically documented (24%), possible and doubtful infections (38%). The classification of infections among the partecipating centres did not differ significantly at least for the 4 centres which provided most of the recorded cases (Roma, Perugia, Bergamo, Genova). No differences were found among centres as far as the microbiologically documented infections are concerned; in fact gram-positive organisms represented the most frequently isolated pathogens in all centres.

TABLE 1. PATIENT CHARACTERISTICS

Febrile episodes (pts)	269	(232)
Mean age (range) yrs	33.3	(1 to 84)
Males/Females	127/105	
Diagnosis		
Acute leukemia	156	(58%)
Lymphoma	31	(12%)
Other	41	(15%)
Bone Marrow Transplantation	41	(15%)
Autologus 21		
Allogeneic 20		
Initial Granulocyte count		
<100 / mmc	134	(49.8%)
100-499/mmc	97	(36%)
500-1000/mmc	23	(8.6%)
> 1000	8	(3%)
Unknown	7	(2.6%)
Protective environment		
Single room	171	(63.5%)
LAFR	23	(8.7%)
Other	17	(6.3%)
No protection	58	(21.5%)
Antinfective prophylaxis	175	(65.3%)
Central Venous Catheter	104	(38.7%)
Fever occuring after hospitalization	210	(78%)
Shock at onset	7	(2.6%)

We focused our analysis on bacteremic episodes. Pathogens responsible for the 91 bacteremias (see Table 2) were in the majority gram-positive (56%) followed by gram-negative bacilli (32%) and fungi (4 %). Seven polymicrobial sepsis were also observed, caused mainly by staphylococci and gram-negative bacilli.

TABLE 2. SEPSIS : BLOOD ISOLATES

STAPHYLOCOCCI	23	(25%)
STREPTOCOCCI	18	(20%)
PNEUMOCOCCI	3	(3%)
ENTEROCOCCI	2	(2%)
OTHER GRAM-POSITIVE ORGANISMS	5	(5%)
TOTAL GRAM-POSITIVE	51	(56%)
E. COLI	15	(16%)
PS. AERUGINOSA	8	(9%)
OTHER GRAM-NEGATIVE BACILLI	6	(6%)
TOTAL GRAM-NEGATIVE	29	(32%)
CANDIDA	4	(4%)
POLYMICROBIAL	7	(8%)
GRAND TOTAL	91	(100%)

This pattern of blood isolates is similar to that found in the most recent E.O.R.T.C. trial (E.O.R.T.C. 1987).
The analysis of pathogens isolated from patients receiving or not oral antibacterial prophylaxis is shown in Table 3.
Patients receiving prophylaxis exhibited a greater percentage of gram-positive blood isolates (66%) in respect to those not receiving prophylaxis (26%). Gram-negative bacilli were instead largely prevalent among patients not receiving prophylaxis (61% vs. 22%). Fungi were isolated only from patients receiving prophylaxis.

TABLE 3. SEPSIS : COMPARISON BETWEEN PATIENTS WITH OR WITHOUT ANTIBACTERIAL PROPHYLAXIS

BLOOD ISOLATES	PATIENTS RECEIVING ORAL PROPHYLAXIS	
	YES *	NO
GRAM-POSITIVE	45 (66%)	6 (26%)
GRAM-NEGATIVE	15 (22%)	14 (61%)
FUNGI	4 (6%)	-
POLYMICROBIAL	4 (6%)	3 (13%)
TOTAL	68 (100%)	23 (100%)

* (Quinolones 63%, Co-trimoxazole 29%)

The overall mortality during bacteremic episodes is shown in Table 4. The highest percentage of deaths was found in patients with fungemia (3/4; 75%) followed by those with sepsis caused by gram-positive organisms (12/51; 23%), gram-negative bacilli (5/29; 17%) and polymicrobial infections (1/7; 14%). However, if one take in account only the deaths due to infection according to investigator's judgment, the mortality rate was greater in patients with gram-negative sepsis. This findings suggests great caution in interpreting data on mortality provided by some studies.

The deaths in bacteremic episodes seems to be directly related to the duration of neutropenia prior to sepsis but no relationship was found with the duration of hospitalization prior to sepsis (Whimbley, 1987).

TABLE 4. SEPSIS : MORTALITY BY PATHOGENS

Pathogens	Total deaths	Deaths due to infection
GRAM-POSITIVE	12/51 (23%)	4/51 (8%)
GRAM-NEGATIVE	5/29 (17%)	4/29 (14%)
FUNGI	3/4 (75%)	3/4 (75%)
POLYMICROBIAL	1/7 (14%)	1/7 (14%)
TOTAL	21/91 (24%)	12/91 (13%)

As might be expected, shock at onset of bacteremic episodes was accompanied by a high mortality (2/4; 50%) and both the deaths occurred in patients with gram-positive sepsis (streptococci).

Empiric antibiotic therapy was started at the beginning of all febrile episodes (269) and was represented mainly by : a beta-lactam plus an aminoglycoside (76%); a beta-lactam plus an aminoglycoside plus an antistaphylococcal agent (15%) and monotherapy with a beta-lactam antibiotic (9%).

The initial therapy was modified during the first febrile episode within 72/96 hours in 50% of patients receiving monotherapy, in 25% of patients receiving double association therapy, in 48% of patients receiving triple association therapy.

Empiric antibiotic therapy is usually modified on the basis of the initial microbiological data and clinical evaluation; however from our data the modifications of antimicrobials seems to be mainly directed by the initial choice of antibiotics : patients receiving an initial beta-lactam monotherapy added mainly an aminoglycoside, those receiving an initial double association added mainly an antistaphylococcal agent and those receiving a triple association added mainly an antifungal agent.

CONCLUSIONS

The above preliminary data refers to the first prospective study on the epidemiology of infection in neutropenic patients at some italian institutions and new information will be provided when the enrollment of patients continues to increase steadily.

The analysis of the first recorded 269 febrile episodes shows that our epidemiological findings are similar to those found in other large international trials. A multivariate analysis of the data would provide more information and understanding on the most important characteristics of the infections in neutropenic patient in our Institutions.

REFERENCES

Inagaki, J.; Rodriguez,V.; Bodey G.P. (1974): Causes of death in cancer patients. Medical and Pediatric Oncology, 5, 241-244.

Whimbley, E.; Kiehn, T.E.; Blevins, A.; Armstrong, D. (1987): Bacteremia and fungemia in patients with neoplastic disease. Am. J. Med., 82, 723-730.

EORTC International Antimicrobial Therapy Cooperative Group (1987): Ceftazidime combined with a short or long course of amikacin for empirical therapy of Gram-negative bacteremia in cancer patients with granulocytopenia. N. Engl. J. Med., 317:1692-1698.

Infections in hematologic patients : 10 years of experiences

A. Chierichini, S. Nardelli, L. Deriu

Divisione di Ematologia, Ospedale S. Maria Goretti, 04100 Latina, Italy

---

ABSTRACT

The incidence of septic episodes in patients affected by hematological malignancies and the results obtained with selected antibiotic associations are analized. All the patients included had severe neutropenia (PMN 1000/mmc) and received prophylactic treatment against bacterial and micotic agents.

KEYWORDS

Hematologic malignancies, severe neutropenia, septic episodes, antibiotic associations.

INTRODUCTION

Between December 1976 and December 1986, we have registred 1294 admissions of patients affected by hematologic malignancies. The median admission rate was 148/years (range 80-204). The diagnosis at admission for all the years were: Acute Leukemias and dismielopoiesis 460; Non Hodgkin and Hodgkin Lymphomas 380; Myeloproliferative disease 154; Chronic Lymphocytic Leukemia 130; Myeloma 140; Bone marrow Aplasia or Ipoplasia 30.
We have analized the incidence of septic episodes and the results obtained with selected antibiotic association.

PATIENTS AND METHODS

All the patients included had a severe neutropenia (PMN 1000/mmc) and received at admission prophylactic treatment against bacterial and micotic agents. (Tab.1).
At onset of fever (38°C and persisting more then 24 H), or in presence of clinical or radiologic evidence of infection, we started

antibiotic therapy after cultural samples(blood,urine,sputum,ecc.).
During teh years we have studied some selected antibiotic associations (Tab 2) that were somministred till clinical or microbiological signs of infections disappeared,or till evidence of resistance.

RESULTS and COMMENTS

The results obtained with each association are shown in Tab.3.
We illustred the sites more frequently involved by the infections in Tab.4 and the frequence of bacteria recovered in Tab.5.
We have summarized the microbic prevalence during the years of investigation:

GRAM + : 1977-1979 Diplococcus Pneumoniae
         1980- 1982 Staphilococcus Aureus and Epidermidis
         1983-1986 Staphilococcus Aureus and Epidermidis
GRAM - : All the years Pseudomonas Aeruginosa
                      Escherichia Coli
                      Klebsiella Pneumoniae

We have had a very low incidence of sepsis (0,5%) and sistemic micosis (1%).
On the contrary ,about 60% of the patients developed oral candidosis expecially during intensive chemotherapy.

REFERENCES

Cohen J.(1984):Empirical antifungal therapy in neutropenic patients.
    J Antimicrob Chemother 13:109-11
Gaya H.(1984)Rational basis for choice of regimens for empirical therapy of sepsis in granulocytopenic patients.
    Clin Hematol 13:573-86
Young L.S.(1986):Empirical antimicrobial therapy in the neutropenic host.N Eng J Med 315:380-81
Marcus E.R.,Goldman J.M?(1986):Management of infection in neutropenic patient.Br Med J 293 :406-8
Pizzo P.A.,Hathorn J.W.,Hicmenz J. et al.(1986):A randomized trial comparing ceftazidime alone with combination antibiotic therapy in cancer patients with fever and neutropenis. N Eng J Med 315: 558-58
Starke I.D.,Donnely J.P.,Catowsky D. et al.(1982):Cotrimoxazole alone for the prevention of bacteria infection in patients with acute leukemia. Lancet ii 5-6

Table 1. PROPHILACTIC SCHEDULE

Bacterial infection: 1976-1983 Trimethoprim 640 mg/die p.o.
                                Sulfametossazolo 3200 mg/die p.o.
                      1984-1986 Norfloxacin 1600 mg/die p.o.
Mycotic infection: 1976-1979 Nystatin topic
                      1980-1984 Amphotericin B 3g/die p.o.
                      1985-1986 Ketoconazole 400mg/die p.o.

Table 2. SELECTED ANTIBIOTIC ASSOCIATIONS

Cefoxitine 150 mg/kg/die + Tobramicin 5 mg/kg/die X 4 doses (A)
Cefotaxime 150 mg/kg/die + Amikacin 15 mg/kg/die   X 4 doses (B)
Ceftazidime 150 mg/kg/die + Amikacin 15 mg/kg/die X 4 doses   (C)
Aztreonam   150 mg/kg/die + Netilmicin 6 mg/kg/die X 4 doses* (D)
              * only in Gram - documented infection

Table 3. CLINICAL FINDINGS AND RESULTS

	A	B	C	D
Septic Episodes	35	35	55	21
Patients cured	14 (40%)	23 (65%)	38 (70%)	15 (71%)
Antibiotic Th.(median d.)	7,5	8	8	9
Absolute PMN count/mmc	336	500	450	500

Table 4. INFECTION INVOLVED SITES

	A	B	C	D
Respiratory tract	21	20	32	11
UTI	4	1	7	1
Soft tissues	5	5	8	3
Sepsis	1	2	0	0
FUO	4	7	8	6

Table 5. BACTERIA

	A	B	C	D
Diplococcus Pneumoniae	4	4	8	0
Streptococcus Hemoliticus	1	0	1	0
Strepyococcus Viridans	5	3	3	0
Enterococcus	1	2	2	0
Staphilococcus A. and E.	4	2	6	0
Klebsiella Pneumoniae	3	0	6	3
Pseudomonas Aeruginosa	5	1	3	0
Salmonella Tiphi	1	0	0	0
Pseudomonas Putida	1	0	1	1
Escherichia Coli	5	2	4	2
Serratia Marcescens	2	0	2	0
Enterobacter Aerogenes	1	0	1	0

Infectious complications in acute leukemic adults : a 4-year retrospective analysis

C. Rinaldi, U. Venturelli[1]

Istituto di Patologia Medica, Università degli Studi di Trieste, [1] Istituto Immunotrasfusionale, O.C. di Udine, Italy

All the febrile episodes occurring in 31 adults with acute leukemia during a 4-year period were reviewed. There was an average of 2.7 febrile episodes/patient and the patients spent 22 per cent of their days in hospital with fever. We documented 82 episodes of fever: 33 MDI, 8 CDI and 41 FUO. Fever occurred most often (72 per cent of cases) when patients had neutropenia (less than 0.5×10^9/L neutrophils). Staphylococcus epidermidis and Escherichia Coli were the predominant pathogens accounting respectively for 32 and 27 per cent of the isolates.

KEY WORDS

Acute leukemia, infectious complications.

INTRODUCTION

Infection remains the major cause of death and morbidity in patients with acute leukemia. In dealing with current status and future prospects for prevention and treatment of infections it is of paramount importance to understand the origin and nature of the responsible organisms and to identify factors which increase the risk of infectious complications. In order to obtain such data we have retrospectively examined all the febrile episodes which occurred in patients affected by acute leukemia during a 4-year period.

MATERIALS AND METHODS

Patients
From July 1983 trough July 1987 31 patients with a diagnosis of acute leukemia were admitted to the Institute of Patologia Medica of Trieste. All periods of hospitalization, from first admission until death or until July 1987 were reviewed.

Classification of febrile episodes

A febrile episode was defined as three temperature elevations exceeding 38°C during a 24-hour period or as a single elevation above 38.5°C.
Each episode of fever was classified according to clinical data, clinical course and microbiology.
Microbiologically documented infections (MDI) were defined as febrile episodes accompanied by clinical signs and symptoms of infection in which a pathogenic organism was recovered.
Clinically documented infections (CDI) were defined as episodes in which signs and symptoms of infection were present but no pathogen was recovered.
Febrile episodes in which no infectious aetiology could be demonstrated were considered fevers of unknown origin (FUO).

Neutrophil count

The neutrophil count at the onset and at the final outcome of each febrile episode was recorded. Neutropenia was defined as a neutrophil count less than $0.5 \times 10^9/L$.

RESULTS

Thirty one patients were included in this analysis (Table 1): 19 males and 12 females; their median age was 54 years (range 19-84).
The underlying disease wan ANLL in 25 patients and ALL in 6.
During the reviewed period the patients spent a total of 2248 days in hospital; 22 per cent of the days were spent with fever, 44 per cent with neutropenia.
Eightytwo episodes of fever were documented: 41 of infectious origin (33 MDI and 8 CDI) and 41 FUO.
The mean duration of fever was 5.9 days (range 1-43): we observed a significative difference between infections (7.2 d.) and FUO (4.8 d.) (P=0.06)

Table 1. Patient characteristics

N. of patients	31
Age (years) : median (range)	54,(19-84)
Sex (males/females)	19/12
ANLL	25
ALL	6
Febrile episodes	82
Duration of fever : mean (range)	5.9 (1-43)
FUO	41
CDI + MDI	41

The incidence of fever was related to the level of circulating neutrophils (Table

2) 59/82 episodes occurred in neutropenic patients and nearly all the most serious infections (including the lethal ones) when neutrophils were less than 0.1×10^9L. Mean duration of fever was longer in cases with severe neutropenia at the onset. However we found no correlation between resolution of fever and granulocyte recovery; in fact in the majority of cases (50/59) patients were still neutropenic when fever resolved.

Table 2. Relationship between fever and degree of neutropenia

NEUTROPHIL COUNT 1×10^9/L	FEBRILE EP. N°	(%)	FEVER DURATION Mean	(Range)
Inf. 0.1	43	(52)	6.3	(1-43)
0.1 - 0.5	16	(20)	4.7	(2-16)
0.5 - 1.0	5	(6)	4.4	(2- 7)
Sup. 1.0	18	(22)	7.2	(2-12)

We observed that incidence of febrile episodes was higher during active phase of the disease (diagnosis, induction, relapse), while patients with ANLL and ALL in complete remission remained mostly free of fever.

Septicemia was by far the most common type of infection (29 episodes) followed by pneumonia (4 cases), soft tissue and urinary tract infections. (Table 3) Of concern is the fact that in the four episodes of pulmonary involvement no infecting organism was isolated in the sputum or in the transtracheal samples.

Table 3. Sites of infection

	MDI	CDI
Septicaemia	29	-
Pneumonia	-	4
Urinary tract	4	-
Skin	-	2
Liver (abscesses)	-	1
Peripheral vein	-	1

The aetiologic agent was identified in 33 febrile episodes (MDI): Gram negative bacilli were the most common phatogens (16 cases) followed by Gram positive organisms (11 cases) and by fungi (4 infections, all caused by Candida species); in 2 episodes both Gram neg. and Gram pos. agents were isolated. Staphylococcus epidermidis and Escherichia Coli were the predominant pathogens accounting respectively for 32 per cent and 27 per cent of the isolates (Table 4).

Table 4. Organisms causing infections

AGENT	N° OF ISOLATES	%
Staph. epidermidis	12	32.4
Staph. saprophyticus	1	2.7
Strepto. alpha hae.	1	2.7
E. Coli	10	27.0
P. aeruginosa	3	8.1
Enterobacter	3	8.1
Klebsiella	2	5.4
Proteus	1	2.7
Candida species	4	10.8

In all Gram positive and multiple agent infections (13 cases) coagulase negative Staphylococci were isolated. The incidence of such agents increased year by year in the reviewed period and this was associated with an increase in the use of long term indwelling catheters. S. Epidermidis and S. saprophitycus isolates showed a wide range of resistance to antimicrobial agents including methicillin and third generation cephalosporins, but they were uniformly susceptible to vancomycin that was the drug of choise. Catheter removal was necessary only in 3 patients, while in the other episodes antibiotic therapy was sucessful without removing the catheter, even if signs of exit site infection were present.

Eleven patients died in the hospital during the reviewed period; in seven cases death was related to documented or possible infections.

DISCUSSION

This study confirms that, despite infection prevention programs (Hann, 1984) the clinical course of patients affected by acute leukemia is still complicated by fever and infections.

In our series there was an average of 2.7 febrile episodes/patient and the patients spent 22 per cent of their days in the hospital with fever. Fever appeared to be a near inevitable consequence of neutropenia since 72 per cent of the episodes occurred in patients with less than 0.5×10^9/L circulating neutrophils. Fifty per cent of the febrile episodes were microbiologically or clinically documented infections, the remaining fifty per cent were considered FUO.

It is likely that a substantial proportion of FUO were actually due to infections. In fact patients with impaired host defenses often fail to develop clini-

cal signs and symptoms of infection. Moreover prompt institution of antibiotic therapy may have resulted in rapid resolution of infection before the diagnosis could be established.
Some viral infections may have been considered FUO since serological studies and viral cultures were not obtained routinely.

During the reviewed period (4-years) we observed a change in the spectrum of organisms causing infections.
The proportion of Gram positive agents increased year by year. The rising incidence of Staphylococcal bacteremia was associated with a greater use of long term indwelling catheters (Hughes ,1985). This changing trend has been noted elsewhere (Winston, 1986; Schiffer, 1987).
The frequency of Staphylococcal infections and the high level of antimicrobial resistance demonstrated by this agent has prompted a renewed interest in the use of a gram positive specific antibiotic (vancomycin) as part of the initial empiric regimen. We think that such terapy is not necessary and not appropiate. In fact vancomycin is costly and a cause of synergistic renal and oto toxicity when combined with aminoglycosides. Moreover Staphylococcal infections produce moderate morbidity but up to date there has been low mortality (in our series 2/13 cases, both of them were multiple agent infections).

REFERENCES

Hann, I.A. (1984) : Infection prophylaxis in the patient with bone marrow failure. Clin Haematol 13,3:523-543
Hughes, C.B. (1985) : Venous access in chemotherapy patients. Iss Oncol 2:4-5
Schiffer, C.A. (1987) : Supportive care: issues in the use of blood products and treatment of infections. Semin Oncol 14,4:454-467
Winston, G.H. (1986) : Infection and transfusion therapy in acute leukaemia. Clin Haematol 15,3:873-904.

Infections and haemorrhage in acute leukaemia, T. Barbui, A. Falanga, B. Minetti, S. Gorini, G. Tognoni and M.D. Donati, eds. John Libbey Eurotext, Paris © 1989, pp. 157-161

Leukemias and HIV-infection : a case report and a brief review of literature

L. Minoli, P. Grossi, A. Malfitano, P. Sacchi, E. Brusamolino[1], G. Pagnucco[1]

Infections Disease and [1] Hematology Depts, University of Pavia, IRCCS San Matteo, Pavia, Italy

RIASSUNTO

All'infuori del Sarcoma di Kaposi, i tumori osservati in corso di infezione da HIV sono rappresentati prevalentemente da forme emolinfoproliferative, in particolare da Linfomi non-Hodgkin e da un minor numero di casi di Morbo di Hodgkin. Complessivamente rara risulta l'osservazione di Leucemie HIV-associate, essenzialmente Leucemie Acute Linfatiche ed eccezionale e' la descrizione di Leucemie non-Linfatiche. La deviazione neoplastica del compartimento linfatico in presenza dell'HIV riconosce fondamenti patogenetici in riarrangiamenti genici e nella deficitaria sorveglianza immunitaria condizionata dal retrovirus con conseguente iperproliferazione linfocitaria ed emergenza di eventuali cloni B-cellulari trasformati. La trasformazione tumorale mieloide e' riconducibile alla dismielopoiesi che precocemente accompagna l'infezione da HIV. Sul piano clinico i tumori HIV-correlati si caratterizzano per una maggior aggressivita', per una minore responsivita' al trattamento e per una piu' elevata frequenza di complicanze infettive.
Gli Autori hanno osservato un caso di Leucemia Acuta HIV-associata morfologicamente ed immunologicamente inquadrabile nel sottotipo L3 FAB. Il decorso clinico non ha presentato peculiarita' rispetto alla corrispondente forma non HIV-associata. Lo studio di laboratorio, peraltro, ed in particolare l'inquadramento bio-immunologico del caso, ha costituito lo spunto di speculazioni patogenetiche.

KEYWORDS: LEUKEMIAS, HIV-INFECTION

INTRODUCTION

Since early descriptions, opportunistic illness observed in the Acquired Immunodeficiency Syndrome has appeared to range in a wide spectrum of infections and fewer malignancies. Among the latter ones, besides Kaposi's Sarcoma, non-Hodgkin Lymphomas and,

less frequently, Hodgkin's disease are described.
HIV-associated leukemias occur rarely and they are almost exclusively Acute Lymphoblastic Leukemias (ALL), often classifiable as FAB L3 (Burkitt-like) subtype. Indeed it is very difficult to distinguish sharply a primitive leukemia from peripheral and bone marrow lymphomatous involvement. Anyway the question is merely theoretical since biological features of both disease are quite similar. Very rare cases of HIV-associated non-lymphoid acute leukemias have been reported, nosology of which, not yet pointed out, could be interpreted as the progression of dismyelopoiesis often encountered in HIV-infected patients.
Generally HIV-associated tumors are characterized by unusual features of localization (e.g. primary CNS lymphoma), aggressive clinical course and scant responsiveness to usual antiblastic chemotherapy.
Cytogenetic techniques applied to investigation of HIV-related tumors have supplied a remarkable contribute to etiopathogenetical deepening of oncology.

CASE REPORT

On April 1987 a 45-year-old male was admitted with fever and purpura. His history was suspect for promiscuous sexual life-style and homosexual intercourses. No relevant previous illness was recorded. Laboratory work-up showed thrombocytopenia, light anemia and peripheral and bone marrow leukemic blast cells, large sized with vacuolized hyperbasophilic cytoplasm, identified as FAB L3 ALL (Burkitt-like) blasts. Blast cell immunological pattern was highmarked by: Ia ++, sIg +++, B4 ++; B1 ++, IgM ++. 8;14 chromosomal translocation was also detected. Search for antibody to Epstein Barr Virus was positive as well as search for antibody to HIV, carried out by testing both blood and CNS fluid.
Remission induction chemotherapy by Vincristine, Daunorubicine, Cyclophosphamide and Prednisone was immediately undertaken, succeeding in complete remission. Intensification sequential courses of high-dose Methotrexate, high-dose Aracytine, m-Amsacrine, Etoposide were twice administered, aside with local prophylactic treatment to CNS. No relevant side effects to treatment were recorded. Clinical and hematological remission lasted for 11 months until march 1988, when, heralded by fever, arthralgias, thrombocytopenia and peripheral blast cells were again detected. Marrow check confirmed leukemic relapse by displaying 50% substitution for blast cells. These were similar to those encountered at onset so to be assigned to FAB L3 subtype, but they were lightly more undifferentiated, sharing the following immunological pattern: Ia +++, sIg ++, B4 +-, B1 +++, IgM +++.
Patient's clinical status worsened rapidly due to progressive anemia, hemorrhages and renal failure. Despite salvage treatment by Mitoxantrone and cure of renal failure the patient underwent exitus on 7th day with DIC.
During the whole illness no major opportunistic infections were recorded. Only relapsing protracted oropharingeal candidosis and HSV-1 gingivostomatitis were observed. Autopsy was not performed.

DISCUSSION

Most hematological tumors reported in HIV-infected patients are high-grade, undifferentiated, B-cell derived non-Hodgkin's Lymphomas. A few cases of HIV-associated Burkitt-like leukemias are tightly related with NHL in a biological settlement.
Recently a peripheral T-cell lymphoma has been described in a patient with AIDS. Furthermore at least two cases of acute myeloblastic leukemia and HIV infection are known to have occurred. Such a rapid review of literature raises a number of pathogenetical questions. With regard to high incidence of B-lineage derived lymphomas and leukemias in AIDS, two factors triggering B-cell neoplastic proliferation are recognizable: HIV and EBV infection. Indeed HIV is known to cause by itself proliferation of B-lymphocytes and, in some animal tumors, retroviral genome has been found to be involved in activating oncogenes. Generally T-cell disfunction, due to HIV, should imply a deficient immune surveillance, responsible for a lymphocyte proliferation and emergency of transformed B-cell clones.
Finding of EBV sequences in the tumors suggests a role of this virus in the pathogenesis of AIDS related B-cell lymphomas. Moreover genic rearrangements, which are often associated with chromosomal abnormalities encountered in Burkitt's lymphomas, cause a derepression of c-myc accounting for B-cell clone neoplastic proliferation. As to the AIDS-associated T-cell lymphoma, Watcher et al suggest that repeated stimulation of T-cell lineage by a number of antigens, unique of such illness, would allow dismission of lymphokines and consequent triggering of T-cells. On the other hand deficient immune system would not be able to remove any malignant clone emerging in the setting of lymphocyte hyperproliferation.
Some more interesting data are supplied by immunological merkers of leukemic blast cells. In fact Burkitt cells are known to express a membrane receptor to IgM, which is tightly related to c-myc expression.
Lastly, occurence of myeloblastic acute leukemia in HIV-infected patients is less comprehensible as to pathogenesis. Anyway progression of myelodysplasia to AML reported by Napoli et al is strongly suggestive for a pathogenetic linkage between myelodysplasia, often encountered in HIV-patients, and emergency of the tumor. Such data are supported by observations of D'Onofrio et al, who have reported dysgranulopoiesis features (peroxidase positive neutrophils and macrocytosis) in peripheral blood of AIDS-patients.
From a clinical point of view HIV-associated lymphomas and leukemias share a worse prognosis due to increased incidence of opportunistic infections linkable to retroviral infection and less responsiveness to antiblastic treatment.
Our case is seemed to be worth mentioning in view of whole rarity of HIV-associated leukemias. Observed clinical course does not share features of severeness, compared with the same hematological disease occuring in HIV-seronegative subjects. Particularly, illness has not been complicated by major opportunistic infections, save but minor Candida and HSV infetions, which usually overlay antiblastic chemotherapy. Treatment courses have not been delayed by pancytopenia and complete remission lasted for a longer time then observed average. Probably the choice of aggressive therapy regimen, tailored to encountered leukemic pattern and employing

sequentially all major antiblastic drugs has allowed to obtain and maintain complete remission for a relatively long time.

With regard to biological features, finding of serum antibody to EBV and 8;14 chromosomal translocation aggrees with observations of literature and confirms above pathogenetical hypothesis. Immunological markers suggestive for B-cell lineage, have ascertained morphological identification of leukemic blast cells and at relapse they have pointed out diagnosis by sharing further cell anaplasia.

In conclusion the whole number of informations supplied in our case by immunobiological investigations, aside with hematological routinary work-up, has allowed us to deepen diagnosis, in order to plan the treatment. It represents a little contribute to knowledge of this illness. Moreover it may be suggested as a model of approaching to the patients with HIV-infection and blood tumor.

RESUME

Outre le Sarcome de Kaposi, les tumeurs que sont observées plus fréquemment lors d'une infection HIV sont représentées par des formes émo-lymphoproliferatives, en particulier des Lymphomes non-Hodgkin et moins fréquemment des cas de maladie de Hodgkin. Dans l'ensemble, on a observé tres rarement leucémies HIV-associées, essentiellement Leucémies Aigües Lymphatiques et exceptionnellement Leucémies non-lymphatiques. La pathogénèse de la déviation neoplastique du compartiment lymphatique, en présence de HIV, peut être en partie attribuée à un déficit de la surveillance immunitaire conditionnée par le rétrovirus; ce qui entraine par conséquence une iperprolifération lymphocitaire et une predominante apparition de clones B-cellulaires transformées.

La transformation cancéreuse myéloide est attribuable à la dy-smyélopoièse qui accompagne trés rapidement l'infection HIV. Au point de vue clinique, les tumeurs HIV-correlées présentent une aggressivité majeure, une mineure sensibilité au traitement et une remarquable fréquence des complications infectieuses.

Les Auteurs ont observé un cas de Leucémie Aigüe HIV-associé morphologiquement et immunologiquement encadrée dans les sous-type FAB-L3. Le suivis clinique a été semblable à celui de la forme non HIV-associé. L'étude de laboratoire, et en particulier l'encadrement bio-immunologique du cas, a constitué l'occasion de spéculations étiopathogenetiques.

REFERENCES

1) Kaplan M H, Susin M, Pahwa S G et al. Neoplastic complications of HTLV III infection. Lymphomas and solid tumors. Am J Med 1987; 82: 389-196.

2) Napoli V M, Stein S F, Spira T J, Raskin D. Myelodysplasia progressing to acute myeloblastic leukemia in an HTLV III virus-positive homosexual man with AIDS-related complex. Am J Clin Pathol 1986; 86: 788-791.

3) Nasr S A, Brynes R K, Garison C P, Chan W C. Peripheral T-cell lymphoma in a patient with Acquired Immune Deficiency Syndrome. Cancer 1988; 61: 947-951.

3) Rechavi G, Ben-Bassat, Berkowicz M et al. Molecular analysis of Burkitt's leukemia in two Hemophilic brothers with AIDS. Blood 1987; 70: 1713-1717.

4) Treacy M, Lai L, Costello C, Clark A. Peripheral blood and bone marrow abnormalities in patients with HIV-related disease. Br J Haematol 1987; 65: 289-294.

5) Willumsen L, Ellegaard J, Pedersen B. HIV-infection in acute myeloblastic leukemia: a similar case. Am J Clin Pathol 1987; 88: 536-537.

Infections and haemorrhage in acute leukaemia, T. Barbui, A. Falanga, B. Minetti, S. Gorini, G. Tognoni and M.D. Donati, eds. John Libbey Eurotext, Paris © 1989, pp. 163-164

Pneumonia caused by legionnaires' disease in a patient with ALL

G. Landonio, R. Cairoli, I. Shlacht[1], I. Errante[1], D. Cipriani

Department of Haematology and Infectious diseases[1], Niguarda-Cà Granda Hospital, Milan, Italy

SUMMARY

We report a case of pneumonia caused by Legionnaires' disease in a patient with ALL treated successfully with the association of eritromicin and rifampicin.

KEY WORDS

ALL, Legionnaires' disease, necrotizing pneumonia with cavitation

INTRODUCTION

Pneumonia caused by Legionnaires' disease bacterium has been documented after exposure to humidifiers and nebulizers. Water storage, distribution system and shower heads have been implicated as Legionella bacteria sources.
Complication include lung abscess and pulmonary fibrosis may occur as a permanent sequela.

CASE REPORT

We report on a 57 y.o. woman affected by ALL treated with standard induction therapy (prednisone, cyclophosphamide, vincristine and daunomycine). On day 17 after starting therapy onset of fever and productive cough. Chest x-ray showed an infiltrate of the superior left lobe. Serology, culture and bronchial brushing were repeatedly negative for mycetes and other microorganism. Fungal pneumonia was suspected and amphotericin B was added to gentamycin and piperacillin. The fever persisted and chest x-ray showed progression of the infiltrate to necrotizing pneumonia with cavitation (fig 1).

Legionnaires' disease was suspected on the base of the x-ray picture. Treatment with other antibiotics was stopped and the patient was started on eriytromycin (2 and after 3 g daily i.v.). Serologic test showed rising titles of specific IgG and IgM. Rifampicin was added to erytromicin (0.9 g dayli p.o.).
The clinical picture improved, the resolution of the infiltrate was, as expected, low.

Figure 1. Chest x-ray presentation on day 24

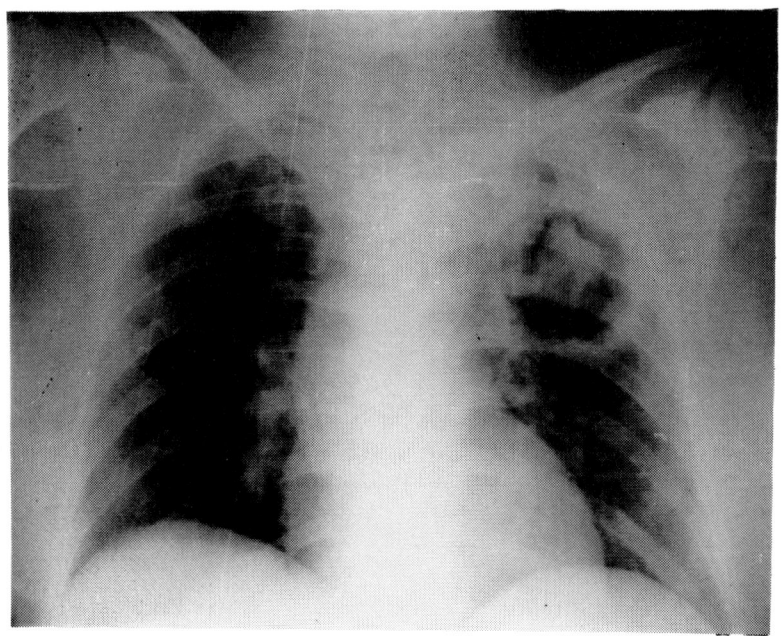

CONCLUSIONS

Lung involvement by Legionnaires' bacterium may be atipical, it must be differentiated from tubercolar or other fungal infections.
Association of erytromycin and rifampicin is an effective treatment. If the use of humidifier is necessary, profilactic measures (steril water etc.) are needed.

REFERENCES

H.Wilczek et al.Nosocomial Legionnaires disease following renal transplantation. Transplantation 1987;43:847-851.

Sonography and percutaneous aspiration of hepatic abscess in a patient with leukemia

L. Cavanna, F. Fornari, G. Civardi, M. Di Stasi, L. Buscarini

[1] Divisione Medica, Ospedale Civile, Via Taverna 49, 29100 Piacenza, Italy

ABSTRACT

A 73 year-old man with chronic lymphocytic leukemia was febrile with recurrence of abdominal pain; a large anechoic mass, consistent with an abscess was disclosed in the liver by ultrasound examination.
The percutaneous abscess drainage was performed using sonography guidance with a fine needle (22 gauge) 15 cm long.
The aspiration yelded 200 ml of pus, cultures demonstrated E. Coli. The patient improved and was discarged, recovered from the abscess 15 days after.
Hepatosplenic infection is an emerging clinical manifestation in patient with hematologic malignancies. Sonography and percutaneous aspiration are quite successful in the diagnosis and tretament of hepatic abscess.

KEYWORDS

Ultrasound, hepatic abscess, leukemia, ultrasonically guided percutaneous aspiration, sonography.

INTRODUCTION

Hepatic abscess is a serious complication of immunocompromised patient. Laboratory data and clinical symptoms are often nonspecific, and the definitive diagnosis may be difficult to establish (Francis 1986). The undrained hepatic abscess causes a reported mortality approaching 100% (Altemeier 1982, Bernardino 1984); modern imaging techniques such as ultrasound (US) and computed tomography (CT), can play an important role in the early diagnosis and treatment of hepatic abscesses (Bernardino 1984).
We report a case of chronic B Lymphocytic leukemia (B CLL) with hepatiq abscess in which US aided in diagnosis and in the guidance of aspiration procedures.

PATIENT AND METHODS

Patient
A 73 year-old man with B CLL stage II diagnosed in 1986 and treated with chlo-

rambucil and prednisone was well until December 1987, when he developed a serious illness, fever and abdominal pain; treatment with antibiotics (ampicillin 3 g daily), was without clinical effect. He was then admitted to our hospital. Physical examination showed aching hepatomegaly, laboratory data revealed elevated ESR (119 mm at the Ist h.), neutropenia (WBC 5,5 X 10^9/l, differential count of 10% neutrophils, 86% lymphocytes, 4% eosinophils), Chest X-ray, ECG were normal. Sonography of the abdomen showed a large anechoic mass with small intra-luminal echoes in the liver parenchima. The echo pattern was consistent with an abscess. The patient was considered a suboptimal surgical candidate because of deteriorated clinical status, then ultrasonically guided percutaneous abscess aspiration was performed using a fine needle (FNB) 0,7 mm (22 gauge) 15 cm long Chiba type

Methods

Scans were performed with a real time linear array scanner in trasverse, longitudinal and oblique planers (Hitachi EUB-26), the percutaneous aspiration was carried out according to the principles previously reported (Buscarini 1985, Fornari 1985) (Before biopsy aspiration, prothrombin assessment and platelet count are mandatory, and their values should be higher than 50% and 70.000/mm^3 respectively). The site of puncture marked on the skin was sterilized and local anesthesia was applied to the abdominal wall; the most convenient route was chosen avoiding the pleura and the great vessels.
The fine needle may be guided either by the free hand technique described by Livraghi (1984), and by ourselves, Buscarini (1985), Cavanna (1987) or by biopsy probes: linear array with a central channel or sector and convex scanner with a lateral apparatus. The needle was guided into the mass, when the needle-tip echo was seen to be in the target (lesion), a 20 ml syringe mounted in a Cameco syringe holder (Cameco Syringe Pistol: Precision Dynamics Company Burbank Ca) was attached and suction applied. When the fluid collection was aspirated, irrigation, of the abscess through the needle was carried out using normal saline and sisomicin 80 mg daily for two time.

RESULTS

Percutaneous puncture of the hepatic lesion performed under US guidance using a 22 gauge needle, produced 200 ml of purulent fluid. Cytology of the fluid showed the presence of cellular debris and distrupted leukocytes. No neoplastic cells were observed. Cultures produced E. Coli.
The patient improved and was discarged, recovered from the abscess 15 days after.

DISCUSSION

Infection is a major cause of morbidity and death in leukemia; the advent of newer cytotoxic drugs and immunosuppressive agents has led to an increase in the incidence of opportunistic infections (Francis 1986).
Intraabdominal abscess can give non specific clinical symptoms and can be clinically confused with other disorders, resulting in a delay in diagnosis with increased morbidity and mortality (Francis 1986, King 1987).

US as well as CT are of value in the detection of hepatosplenic abscess (Francis 1986, King 1987, Pastakia 1988) and can also be utilized to guide interventional procedures for definitive diagnosis and treatment. Despite surgical drainage, mortality rates for liver abscess are still high. Moreover the majority of patients present a dramatic clinical picture leading to high operative mortality rates or inoperability. Percutaneous needle aspiration or drainage techniques have assumed importance with the development of newer imaging methods such as CT and US.

In a series of 180 intraabdominal abscesses treated by US-guided drainage, re-. ported by Nielsen (1988), 85% were cured, and Nielsen (1988) supports that conventional surgical treatment has a few important drawbacks: it is stressing to the patient, time consuming and it contaminates the invironment of the hospital. The US-guided drainage of intraabdominal abscess overcome these problems perfectly.

To conclude, we believe that US should be performed early in all patients with suspected abdominal infections, and when a focal lesion, consistent with an abscess is disclosed, US-guided aspiration procedures are not only of values in the cytological and microbiological diagnosis, but can also be utilized for the treatment of abdominal abscesss.

REFERENCES

- Francis, I.R. et al. (1986): Hepatic abscesses in the immunocompromised patient: role of CT in detection, diagnosis, management, and follow-up. Gastrointestinal Radiology 11, 257-262.
- Bernardino, M.E. et al. (1984): Percutaneous drainage of multiseptated hepatic abscess. Journal Computer Assisted Tomography 8, 38-41.
- Altemeier, W.A. et al. (1982): Abscess of the liver: surgical considerations. Arch. Surg. 101, 258-265.
- Buscarini, L. et al. (1985): Ultrasonically guided fine needle biopsy: a new useful technique in pathological staging of malignant lymphoma. Acta Haemat. 73, 150-152.
- Fornari,F. et al. (1985): Il drenaggio percutaneo ecoguidato di ascessi e raccolte liquide addominali. US. Med. 6, 303-313.
- Livraghi, T. (1984): A simple no-cost technique for real time biopsy. J. Clin. Ultrasound 12, 60-62.
- Cavanna , L. et al. (1987): Ultrasound and ultrasonically guided biopsy in hepatic lymphoma. Eur. J. Cancer Clin. Oncol. 23, 323-326
- King, D J. et al. (1987): Unusual presentation of opportunistic infection in patients with leukemia: identification of fungal lesions by ultrasound. J. Clin. Ultrasound 15, 486-489.
- Pastakia, B. et al. (1988): Hepatosplenic candidiasis: wheels within wheels. Radiology 166, 417-421.
- Nielsen, L. (1988): US guided percutaneous treatment of intraabdominal abscesses. Atti V° Corso Nazionale di Aggiornamento in Ecografia Operativa. Fornari F., Cavanna L., Filice C., eds. Ed. Malvezzi Piacenza, pag. 40.

Febrile and infectious episodes in ANLL patients during induction chemotherapy

E. Orlandi, E. Brusamolino, M. Lazzarino, A. Canevari, E. Morra, G. Castelli, D. Caldera, C. Bernasconi

Divisione di Ematologia, Policlinico San Matteo, IRCCS, Pavia, Italy

We retrospectively analysed the incidence and the outcome of febrile episodes of unknown origin (FUO) and of clinically (CDI) or microbiologically (MDI) documented infections in 86 consecutive patients with "de novo" ANLL after intensive induction chemotherapy. Seventy patients (81.5%) suffered from one or more FUO episodes or infections: 47 FUO, 10 CDI, 17 MDI. The predominant pathogens were Gram-negative organisms. Altogether, in our ANLL patients mortality due to possible or proven infection was 26/86 (30%). About one third of febrile and infectious episodes were responsive to combined antimicrobial therapy. In about one third of the events, the increase in neutrophil count above 0.5×10^9 /L was required to recover from FUO or infection.

KEY WORDS

Acute Non Lymphoid Leukemia Fever Infections

INTRODUCTION

We retrospectively analysed the incidence and the clinical outcome of febrile (FUO) and of clinically (CDI) or microbiologically (MDI) documented infections in 86 patients with Acute Non Lymphoid Leukemia (ANLL), admitted to the Hematology Division of Pavia between January 1985 and March 1988.

PATIENTS AND METHODS

Median age of our evaluable patients was 44 years (range: 18-83) F/M ratio was 38/48. At admission, mean neutrophil count was 1.33×10^9 /L, mean platelet count was 80.34×10^9 /L, mean Hb value was 9.54g/dl. According to the FAB criteria, 34 cases were classified as M0-M2, 21 as M3, 30 as M4-M5 and 1 case as M6. In 45 patients the neutrophil count was $\leq 0.5 \times 10^9$ /L. At admission, 14 patients were febrile (FUO) and 4 patients had documented infections. In these cases induction chemotherapy, was started after the resolution of fever or infectious episode. All patients received intensive remission induction chemotherapy, and the adopted regimens were the following: DNR+ARA-C (29 cases), DNR+ARA-C+VP16 (40 cases), ARA-C+VP16 (12 cases), DNR or IDA (5 cases). Nine patients died during therapy administration. After the first course of therapy, 35 patients entered complete remission, 5 patients achieved partial remission and 11 patients were not responsive. Twenty six patients died during the postinduction aplastic phase. As to the supportive care, routine surveillance cultures were not performed. All patients were treated in conventional rooms and received oral amphotericin B or nystatin as antifungal prophylaxis and cotrimoxazole as selective intestinal decontamination. None of our patients was carrying indwelling intravenous catheter. Empiric antibiotic therapy was promptly started in patients with clinically suspected infection. As first-line empiric antibiotic combination we selected gentamicin+cefotaxime; the subsequent combinations were piperacillin+ amikacin or ceftazidime+aztreonam. Before starting empiric therapy, blood culture, urine culture and additional studies as clinically indicated were undertaken. During febrile or infectious episode, culture from blood and other clinically suspicious site were done. If the pathogen organism was isolated, antibiotics were changed according to the susceptibility testing results. Parentheral amphotericin B was administered if a fungal infection was documented or to patients resistant to antibiotic therapy. Therapeutic granulocyte transfusions were occasionally employed (10 cases).

RESULTS

All evaluable patients (77 cases) showed severe neutropenia ($\leq 0.5 \times 10^9$ /L); in 91% of cases the neutrophil nadir was $\leq 0.1 \times 10^9$ /L. The mean interval from the start of chemotherapy to the neutrophil nadir was 10.5 days ($\pm$ 4.41) and the mean duration of severe neutropenia was 21 days ($\pm$ 11.07). In 7 cases neither fever nor infection was detected. Seventy of 77 patients (91%) became febrile. The mean interval from chemotherapy to fever was 11 days ($\pm$ 4.22) and the mean duration of fever was 8.35 days ($\pm$ 6.41). 81% of the febrile or infectious episodes occurred at neutrophil level $\leq 0.1 \times 10^9$ /L.

Fourty seven episodes of FUO were recorded in 41 patients, 6 patients accounting for 2 episodes each. Eleven patients died during FUO, often terminating in organ failure. Sixteen CDI were observed in 14 patients (2 patients showed 2 simultaneous infectious events); six patients died of infection (1 encephalitis and 5 pneumonias). Fifteen had MDI; 2 patients had cellulitis and sepsis sustained by the same pathogen organism. Five patients died of sepsis. The nature and the etiology of the infectious complications are described in table 1. Bacteremias and pneumonias accounted for 70% of proven infections. In our patients not carrying indwelling catheter, Gram negative bacteria were the predominant isolated.

Altogether, the febrile and infectious episodes evaluable for response to the antibiotic therapy according to trend in neutrophil count were 75 (table 2): 29% were lethal, 36% were responsive to empiric or specific antibiotic therapy, regardless of the trend in neutrophil level and in 35% of the episodes the increase in neutrophil count $\geq 0.5 \times 10^9$/L was required to the clinical improvement. No significant differences were observed among the three event groups (FUO, CDI, MDI). Thirty five of 86 patients died. No events directly related to extrahematologic drug toxicity were observed. In 26/86 patients death was due to proven or suspected infection and in 9 patients was due to severe hemorrhage.

CONCLUSIONS

In our experience, infections remain a relevant cause of morbidity and mortality in extremely neutropenic ANLL patients given intensive induction chemotherapy. In patients not carrying indwelling intravenous catheter Gram negative bacteria were the predominant pathogens. The low incidence of definible infections could be ascribed to the prompt initiation of empiric antibiotic therapy. About one third of febrile and infectious episode were responsive to empiric or pathogen oriented antibiotic therapy, independently of the persistance of severe neutropenia; in about one third of the events, a favorable response required the increase in neutrophil count to more than 0.5×10^9/L in addition to antimicrobial therapy. A rapid bone marrow recovery is a prerequisite for the ultimate improvement in granulocitopenic patients with infections sustained by multiresistant organisms or with undiagnosed nonbacterial infection.

Tabel 1 - TYPE OF INFECTIONS AND ISOLATED ORGANISMS (33 EPISODES)

Infection	CDI N°	MDI N°	Organism	N° (site)
Sepsis	-	11	E. Coli	7 (blood 6) (cellulitis 1)
Pneumonitis	9	3		
Cellulitis/abscess	5	2	Pseudom. Aer	6 (blood 4) (cellulitis 1) (lung 1)
Urinary tract	-	1		
Encephalitis	1	-		
Sinusitis	1	-	Serratia marc.	1 (blood)
			Klebsiella pneum.	1 (lung)
			Enterobacter cl.	1 (urine)
			Aspergillus fum.	1 (lung)

Table 2 - RESPONSE TO EMPIRIC OR PATHOGEN-ORIENTED ANTIBIOTIC THERAPY ACCORDING TO TREND IN NEUTROPHIL COUNT

	N°			
	FUO	CDI	MDI	TOTAL (%)
Evaluable episodes	43	16	16	75
Lethal episodes	11	6	5	22(29)
Response to empiric or specific therapy	17	5	5	27(36)
Response requiring recovery from neutropenia	15	5	6	26(35)

Unusual opportunistic mycoses and concomitant bacteremia in patients with haematological malignancy

B. Minetti, B. Marini, F. Gnecchi[1], C. Farina[2], M.A. Viviani[3], T. Barbui

Divisione di Ematologia, [1] Divisione di Malattie Infettive, [2] Servizio di Microbiologia, Ospedali Riuniti di Bergamo, [3] Istituto di Igiene, Università degli Studi di Milano, Italy

Abstract

Unusual Systemic Fungal Infections (USFI) caused by *Cryptococcus* spp., *Fusarium* spp. and *Geothricum* spp. were found in five compromised haematological patients. USFI diagnosis was based on repeated isolation of pure colonies from blood, CSF and skin specimen cultures. Four of five patients showed a concomitant bacterial septicaemia, thus it seems mandatory looking for fungi, also when a common pathogen organism has been previously isolated.

Introduction

Systemic fungal infection with a net prevalence of *Candida* spp. and *Aspergillus* spp. is an important cause of morbidity and mortality in patients with haematological malignancy, particularly if severely granulocytopenic (Bodey G.P. et al., 1986) and/or treated with high dose corticosteroids (Bennett J.E., 1987).

Recently, Unusual Systemic Fungal Infections (USFI) have been reported, caused by *Cryptococcus neoformans*, *Trichosporon* spp., *Fusarium* spp. and *Geotrichum* spp (Walsh T.J. et al., 1986; Anaissie E. et al., 1986).

Here we report *Cryptococcus neoformans*, *Fusarium proliferatum*, *Fusarium verticilloides* and *Geotrichum capitatum* systemic infections in five haematological patients. Aim of this report is to alert on the possible pathological role of such agents in higly compromised patients.

Patients and methods

Patients:
Five patients with advanced, refractory haematological malignancy, admitted to our Division, receiving aggressive antineoplastic treatment and remaining with a granulocyte count below 0.1×10^9/L for 1-5 weeks, were diagnosed as having USFI. An invasive fungal infection was suspected by clinical manifestations and diagnosis was confirmed on repeated isolation of pure colonies from blood, cerebrospinal fluid and skin specimens cultures. Patients' characteristics at the beginning of the clinical infectious symptoms are summerized in Table 1

Tab. 1: Patients' characteristics at the beginning of the clinical infectious symptoms.

Patients (No)	Age/Sex	Haematological diagnosis	Antineoplastic treatment	Days of severe granulocytopenia*	Days of PDN (>1mg/Kg/d)
1.	53/M	High grade non-Hodgkin lymphoma	CHOP	14	10
2.	54/M	Acute myeloid leukaemia	DAT	15	0
3.	36/M	Refractory acute myeloid leukaemia	DAT	8	10
4.	29/M	Resistent Hodgkin disease	CBV + ABMT	16	12
5.	47/F	Refractory acute lymphoid leukaemia	Cytarabine Etoposide Mitoxantrone	35	28

* Granulocyte count below 0.5×10^9/L

Culture methods:
Blood from all patients was bed-side inoculated into two BACTED-system bottles (6A and 7A), each containing 30 ml of tryptic soy broth (Johnson Lab., Inc, Towson, Md). Gram-stained smears were performed on BACTED bottles if turbidity, haemolisis or gas was observed and if growth indices of 30 or incremental changes in the growth indices of 10 were displayed.
Sample of blood which demostrated blastoconidia (cases 1, 2) or branching hyphae (cases 3-5) at direct microscopical examination were withdrawn from Bactec bottles and 0.1 ml was inoculated onto each of six plates (5% sheep blood, McConkey, Chapman, Chocolate and Sabouraud agars). Bacteriological plates were incubated at 35°C, chocolate agar under 5% CO_2 and Sabouraud plates at 35°C and 30 ° C.
Macroscopic colony characteristics and microscopic examination in lactophenol cotton blue mounts were made from subcultures grown on Sabouraud glucose agar, and identification was according with Barnett et al. (1984).
In case 2 CSF fluid was directly examinates after India-ink preparation to exhibite by a capsular halo around blastospores. In this case, it was also possible to detect a high titer of cryptococcal antigens in serum and in CSF (> 1: 2048) (Crypto-Latex, Bouty SpA, Hata).
In case 5 skin specimens, taken from an area previously cleansed with 70% alcohol and scraped with a scalpel, were cultured onto Sabouraud agar for fungi detection.

Results and discussion
Pertinent clinical and microbiological data for USFI are showed in Table 2 and Table 3, respectively.

Tab. 2 : Clinical data of the patients diagnosed for USFI

Patient (No.)	USFI Symptoms	Culture studies			Treatment and outcome
		Specimens	Positive/Total	Organisms	
1.	Pneumonia	Blood	3/5 5/5	S. pneumoniae C. neoformans	Cefazolin. Death.
2.	Meningo-encephalitis	Blood CNS fluid	3/3 3/9	K. pneumoniae C. neoformans	Ceftriaxone, Amikacin, Rifampin+INI, Fluoro-cytosine. Death
3.	Paralytic ileus	Blood	8/20	Geotrichum capitatum	Piperacillin, Amikacin, Metronidazole, Amphotericin B. Death.
4.	Septicaemia	Blood	11/17	Enterococci, Fusarium proliferatum	Ceftazidime, Amikacin, Vancomycin. Death.
5.	Septicaemia	Blood Skin	4/12 3/12 4/12 4/8	P. aeruginosa Gram+ rods Fuserium verticilloides F. verticilloides	Piperacillin, Amikacin, Amphotericin B. Death.

Tab. 3 Microbiological characteristics of isolated fungi.

Genus/Species	Rate of growth	Colony characteristics*	Microscopic characteristics
Cryptococcus neoformans	Rapid: 3 days.	At first: flat or slighty heaped, shiny, moist, often mucoid colonies, with withish-cream color. Later: brunish	No visible hyphae Capsules in vivo (India Ink Col). Diam: 4-8 um. Blastoconidia.
Geotrichum capitatum	Rapid: 4 days.	At first: white, moist, yeast-like and easily picked-up colonies. Later: short, white, cottony aerial mycelium.	True septate hyphae. Rectangular artroconidia. Diam: 4-10 um.
Fusarium spp.	Rapid: 4 days	At first: cottony and withish colonies. Later: pink, orange or violet with a lighter periphery. Reverse is light in color.	Septate hyphae phialoconidia
F. proliferatum		Microconidia clavate forming long chaines and macroconidia 3-5 septate produced from phialides proliferating sympodially.	
F. verticilloides		Microconidia clavate forming long chaines and macrocinodia almost straighted from phialides proliferating with a single-opening and non-sympodially.	

Four of five patients with haematological malignancy were found to have USFI and a concomitant bacterial septicaemia. USFI diagnosis was based on repeated isolation of pure colonies from blood and cerebrospinal fluid cultures, and on the clinical picture of systemic infecious diseases despite the administration of broad-spectrum antibacterial treatment. Unfortunately, only in 3 of the 5 patients a specific antifungal treatment was done and no clinical response was obtained.

In conclusion this comunication contributes to expand the knowledge of the USFI in patients with haematological malignancy and suggests that a search for fungal infection should be done even in patients with a well established bacterial infection, regardless to the responce of a broad-spectrum antibacterial treatment. This is likely to evaluate the prevalence of USFI in the higly compromised haematological patients, to facilitate a correct diagnosis and beginning of a early and specific treatment.

References

Anaissie E., Kantarjian H., Jones P., Barlogie B., Luna M., Lopez-Berenstain G., Bodey G.P. (1986) A newly recognized fungal pathogen in immunosuppressed patients. Cancer, 57: 2141-2145.

Barnett J.A., Payne R.W., Yerrow D.(1983) Yeast: characteristics and identification. Cambridge University Press, Cambridge.

Bennett J.E. (1987) Fungal infections. In Harrison's Principles of Internal Medicine, 11th eds, pp 736-745.

Bodey G.P. (1986) Fungal infection and fever of unknown origin in neutropenic patients. Am. J. Med. 80 (Suppl. C), 112-119.

Walsh T.J., Newman K.R., Mooly M., Wharton R.C., Wade J.C. (1986) Trichosporonosis in patients with neoplastic disease. Medicine, 65: 268-279.

Pulmonary and myocardial infarction secondary to arterial occlusion by *Aspergillus fumigatus* in ANLL

G. Landonio[1], A.M. Nosari[1], L. Gargantini[1], F. De Cataldo[1], P. Oreste[2]

[1] Department of Haematology and [2] Pathology, Ospedale Niguarda Ca' Granda, Milan, Italy

SUMMARY

Invasive aspergillosis is a fulminant and highly lethal infection of severely compromised patients. Hematogenous dissemination produces lesions in almost any organ. Myocardial infarction, though uncommon, has been described in some cases. We report the clinical picture of a patient with ANLL.

KEY WORDS

Aspergillosis, immunocompromised patient, myocardial infarction.

INTRODUCTION

Invasive aspergillosis is a fulminant and highly lethal infection of severely compromised patients, particularly those predisposed by acute leukemia, granulocytopenia, cytotoxic chemotherapy and corticosteroids.
The respiratory tract is the usual portal of entry. Following colonization of the airways, hyphae penetrate through the walls of bronchi or bronchioles into adjacent pulmonary arteries or arterioles. Vascular invasion, with subsequent thrombomycotic occlusion, is responsible for the typical parenchymal lesion of invasive aspergillosis, the nodular infarct. Hematogenous dissemination, another consequence of hyphal angioinvasion, commonly produces lesions in the central nervous system, myocardium, kidneys, gastrointestinal tract, liver and spleen, but almost any organ can be involved.

CASE REPORT

This case concerned a 52 y.o. male patient affected by acute non lymphoblastic leukemia (FAB : M2).
He was treated by standard induction therapy (ARA-C + Daunomycin). WBC nadir ($0.4 \times 10^9/l$) was reached on day 5

after the end of chemotherapy. On day 10 the patient, previously apyretic and asymptomatic, had an episode of acute dyspnea with fever (39 C). Chest X-ray, tomography and pulmonary scintigram were compatible with diagnosis of pulmonary embolism.
The patient was so started on heparin and antibiotic standard regimen (piperacillin + gentamicin). No response by multiple cultures of expectorated sputum and by blood cultures.
The patient showed an apparent clinical improvement, with decrease of fever and dyspnea; WBC: $1.1 \times 10^9/l$; Platelet count: $137 \times 10^9/l$; ECG: normal.
On day 24 the patient had persistent anginal pain with ECG compatible with anterior myocardial infarction.
The patient was transferred to the coronary unit and started on a new antibiotic regimen (ceftriaxone + vancomicin + amikacin + ketoconazole). Chest X-ray showed further worsening of the left lung opacity.
The patient died on day 35, after a down-hill course.

AUTOPSY FINDINGS

Gross examination showed multiple infarction involving the whole left lung, the septal and anterior myocardial walls, the left kidney and spleen.
Histologic examination revealed arterial occlusion due only to intravascular hyphae growth (Aspergillus Fumigatus). Figure 1 shows pulmonary fungal dissemination; figure 2 shows coronary occlusion by hyphae; figure 3 shows hyphae dissemination interesting also myocardial wall.

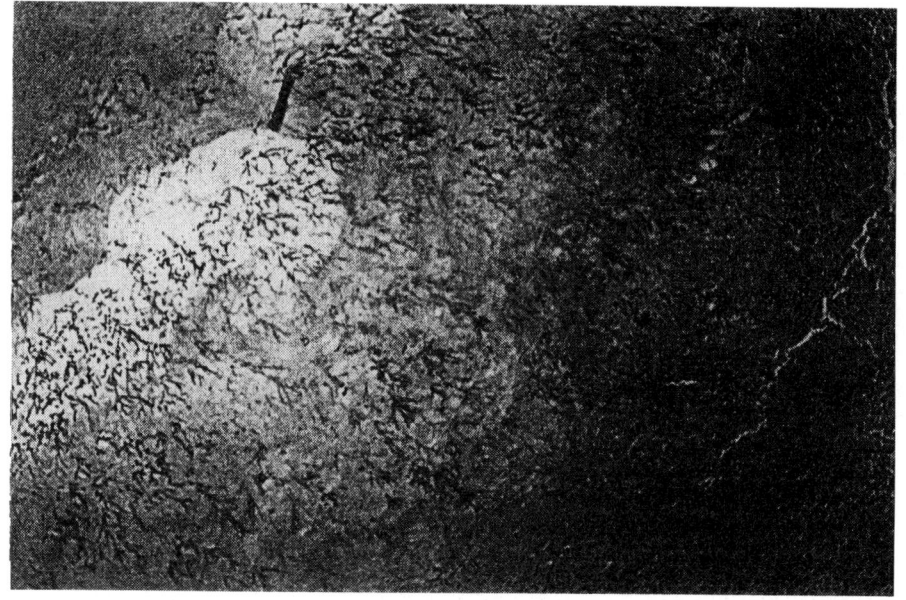

FIG. 1 - Pulmonary dissemination by Aspegillus Fumigatus.

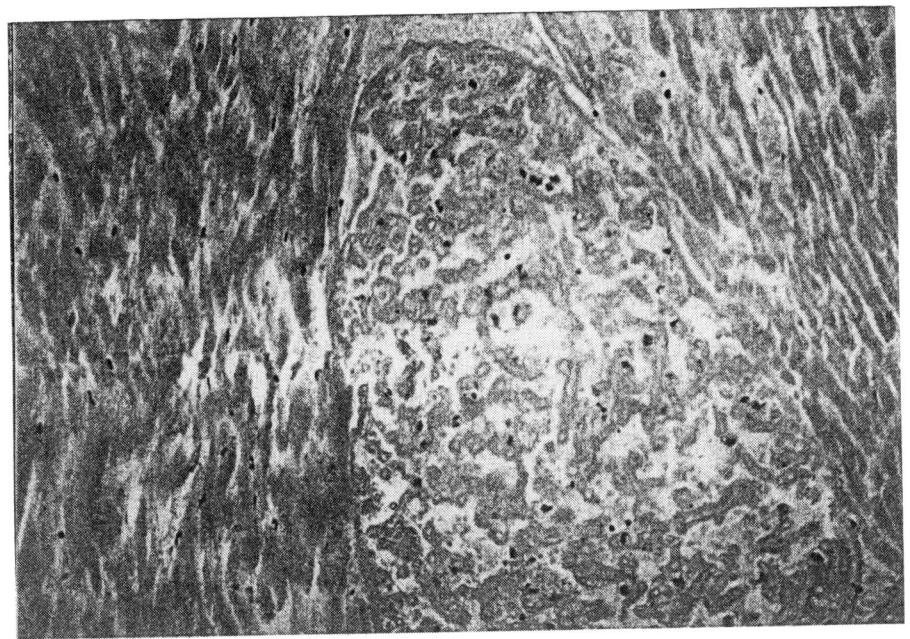

FIG. 2 — Coronary occlusion by hyphae dissemination.

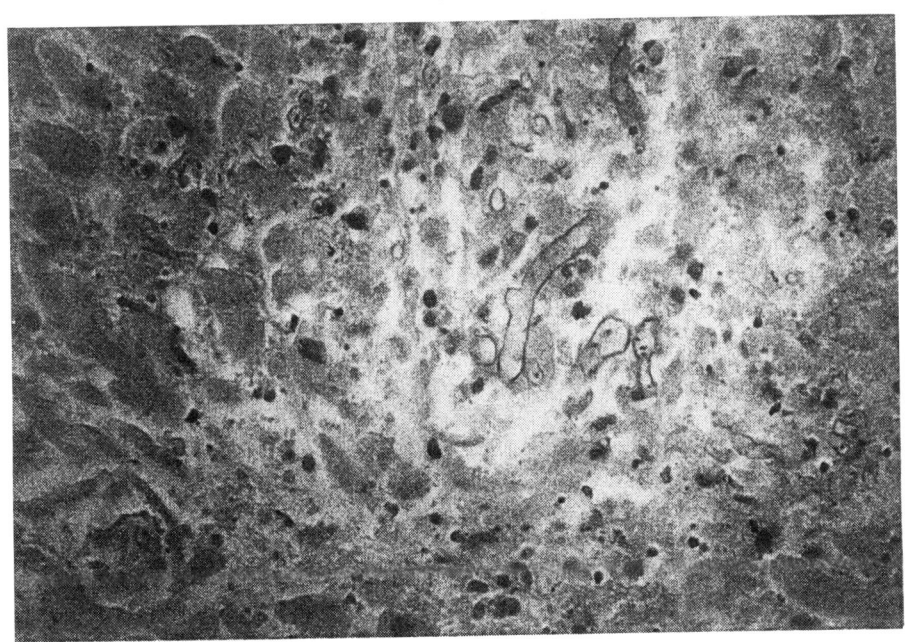

FIG. 3 — Hyphae dissemination interesting myocardial walls.

DISCUSSION

The Aspergillus species are saprophytic moulds of cosmopolitan distribution, and their conidia are ubiquitous within the environment. Of the hundred of recognized species, only about a dozen are genuin human pathogens; species in the Aspergillus Fumigatus, Aspergillus Flavus and Aspergillus Niger groups account for the majority of cases of human aspergillosis.
Aspergillosis is frequently observed in immunocompromised as secondary invasive infection: granulocytopenia, steroid use and cytotoxic drugs are the risk factors recognized in the most number of patients. The infection is characterized by hyphal invasion of blood vessels, thrombosis, necrosis and hemorragic infarction. Clinically these patients show productive cough, dyspnea and fever.
Young et al. (1) reviewed the spectrum of aspergillosis in 98 patients: the vast majority of them had pulmonary lesions, but the x-ray films of the chest may be normal early in the course and become abnormal only later as pulmonary infiltrates evolve. Disseminated disease occurred in a third of the cases; almost half the patients had brain involvement of the kidney, liver and thyroid gland is rather frequent. Nonspecific ST-segment and T-wave changes are the most common ECG abnormalities when the heart is involved. Congestive heart failure may develop in affected patients.
The finding of a true myocardial infarction is uncommon: three only cases in leukemic patients have been described by Andersson et al. (2).
This case emphasizes how much the clinical picture astray and how much the fungal dissemination can be extended.
An incorrect diagnosis was made and no specific treatment was started. Most studies agree with the observation that aspergillosis is frequently recognized at autopsy. However awareness of its possible occurrence and some diagnostic procedures (bronchial brushing, serology and biopsy) might allow an earlier diagnosis in some cases.

REFERENCES

1 .   Young RC, Bennett JE, Vogel CL, et al. Aspergillosis: the spectrum of the disease in 98 patients.
      Medicine. 1970; 49: 147-173.
2 .   Andersson BS, Luna MA, McCredie KB. Systemic aspergillosis as cause of myocardial infarction.
      Cancer. 1986; 58: 2146-2150.

Fatal course of cryptosporidiosis in a case of ANLL (FAB : M3)

A.M. Nosari, A. Freyrie, D. Cipriani, M.R. Villa[1], C. Schiantarelli[1]

Department of Haematology and [1] Infectious Disease, Niguarda Ca' Granda Hospital, Milan, Italy

SUMMARY

Cryptosporidiosis has been described in last years in immuno-compromised and immunocompetent persons. AIDS is the most common underlying illness, but rarely cryptosporidium has been found in cases of acute leukemia. We report the case of a patient who developed cryptosporidiosis in course of induction therapy for ANLL:

KEY WORDS

Cryptosporidiosis, Acute leukemia, induction therapy.

INTRODUCTION

The protozoan parasite Cryptosporidium is increasingly recognized as a cause of enterocolitis in humans (1).
Cryptosporidium, a coccidium, infects the microvillous border of the gastrointestinal tract (from pharynx to rectum) of many animals (mammals, birds, fishes) and humans. Infection may be acquired by conctact with stools of infected animals (35%), trasmission person to person is also possible (65%).
Oocysts have been also detected in bile and respiratory tract secretions.
Human infestations have been considered rare: the first case of human infection was reported in 1976; since then, the number of identified cases substantially increased, because of the recognition of a severe form in patients with AIDS.
In immunocompetent persons (2) Cryptosporidium may cause self-limited gastroenteritis:after a 5 - 14 days incubation-period, nausea, vomiting, low-grade fever, watery diarrhea and crampy abdominal pain lasting few days to weeks, occur.
In contrast,cryptosporidiosis in immunocompromised host (3) is characterized by intractable watery diarrhea, leading to malabsorption and weight loss, that is extremely associated with high mortality.
The acquired immunodeficiency syndrome is the most common underlying illness but cases have also occurred in patients receiving immunosuppressive therapy (acute leukemia, bone marrow

(5) and renal trasplantation (6)) or with congenital hypogammaglobulinemia(7).

CASE REPORT

This case concerned a 52 y.o. female affected by ANLL (FAB:M3)
Induction therapy: standard Daunomycin + ARAC regimen.
WBC nadir $0.1 \times 10/l$ was obtained on day 6 after therapy.
On day 7 the patient developed a diffuse erythematous rash and diarrhea, with fever (39 C) and diffuse abdominal pain.
Stools were positive for staphilococcus pyogenes and candida; negative for enteric pathogens, clostridium, campylobacter, yersinia and parasites.
The patient was treated with vancomicin, imipenem and ketoconazole, without any improvement of the gastroenteric symptoms, despite a concomitant amelioration of the haematologic parameters.
Watery stools became more and more profuse and the patient had an electrolytic and haemodinamic imbalance so marked as to require intensive care treatment.
Here, the patient was examined with colonscopy (day 18) resulted negative for signs of pseudomembranous colitis, and with esophagogastroscopy (day 21) that showed diffuse mucosal candidiasis.
Other tests were unyelding.
Only on day 31 cryptosporidium was searched and found in a stool specimen by a modified Kinyoun stain (8).
The patient died the following day.
Autopsy permis was not granted.

METHODS

Fresh stools or preserved in 2.5% potassium dichromate are concentrated following Rictchie's formalin-diethylacetate sedimentation procedure.
Specimens should be coloured with two methods:1)estemporaneous with Fuchsin-Carbol: mix faces with staining-solution (1/1) and air-dry. Immediate microscopy examination with 40 x is necessary. Refractile and trasparent parasites are shown.
2) permanent with Kinyoun-modified acid-fast stain: oocysts have thick walls, stain pink-red and some contain darkly stained granules (8).

DISCUSSION

The severity of cryptosporidial diarrhea is well illustrated by our patient , died for electrolytic and haemodinamic imbalance,despite the good haematological recovery. In fact fluid and electrolyte therapy and parenteral nutrition have been successfull in sustaining patients for several months,but in these cases also cryptosporidiosis has persisted until death.
Cryptosporidium must be suspected in immunocompromised patients with very profuse watery diarrhea; in fact this infestation has been increasingly documented in this type of patients: there are published records of patients with AIDS or with immunoglobulin deficiency and under immunosuppressive treatment.

In acute lymphoblastic leukemia cryptosporidiosis has been reported so far in two children during maintenance therapy, but not in induction therapy; in our patient the severe agranulocitosis justifies the seriousness of clinical course.
The first cases of human cryptosporidiosis were diagnosed by duodenal or jejunal biopsy.
In recent years some simple and sensitive techniques have been developed for identifying oocysts in stools, including the methods used in our patient.
Antimicrobial treatment for cryptosporidial infection has been singularly unsuccessful in previous reports despite of a variety of potentially active drugs; in addition, the majority of patients received conventional broad-spectrum antibiotics for the treatment of superinfections or suspected sepsis, again without apparent effect on the cryptosporidiosis.
Transient and small improvement were obtained with spiramycin or furazolidone (5-10).
Cryptosporidiosis should be considered always in the differential diagnosis of overwhelming diarrhea in haematological patients with severe immunosuppression.

References

1. Anonymous Cryptosporidiosis (Editorial) Lancet 1984;i:492-493
2. Current WL, Reese NC, Ernst JV, Bailey WS, Heyman MB, Weinstein JM. Human cryptosporidiosis in immunocompetent and immunodeficient persons: studies of an outbreak and experimental trasmission N Eng. J Med 1983;308:1252-7
3. Wolfson JS, Richter JM, Waldron MA, Weber DJ, Mc Carthy DM, Hopkins CC. Cryptosporidium in immunocompetent patients N.Engl. J Med 1985; 312: 1278-82
4. Pitlik SD, Fainstein V, Garza D, Guarda L, Bolivar R, Rios A, Hopfer RL, Mansell PA. Human cryptosporidiosis: Spectrum of Disease Arch. Intern. Med. 1983; 143: 2269-75
5. Collier AC, Miller RA, Meyers JD. Cryptosporidiosis after marrow trasplantation : person-to-person trasmission and treatment with Spiramycin. Ann. Intern. Med. 1984; 101:205-6
6. Weisburger WR, Hutcheon DF, Yardley JH, Roche JC, Hillis WD, Carache P. Cryptosporidiosis in an immunosuppressed renal-trasplant recipient with IgA deficiency. Am. Clin. Pathol. 1979; 72: 473
7. Lasser kh, Lewin kj, Ryning FW. Cryptosporidial enteritis in a patient with congenital Hypogammaglobulinemia. Hum. Pathol.1979;10:234
8. Ma P, Soave R. Three-step tool examination for cryptosporidiosis in ten Homosexual men with protracted watery diarrhea. J Infect. Dis. 1983; 147: 824-8
9. Miller RA, Holmberg RE, Clausen CR. Life-threatening diarrhea caused by cryptosporidium in a child undergoing therapy for acute lymphocytic leukemia J. Pediatr. 1983; 103: 256-9
10. Lewis IJ, Hart CA, Baxby D. Diarrhea due to cryptosporidium in acute lymphoblastic leukemia Arch. Dis. Child. 1985;60:60-2
11. Portnoy D, Whiteside ME, Bukley III E et al. Treatment of intestinal cryptosporidiosis with Spiramycin Ann. Intern. Med. 1984;101: 202-4

The best empiric antibiotic therapy for febrile episodes in patients with acute leukemia

P. Martino, A. Micozzi, G. Gentile, C. Girmenia, R. Raccah, F. Mandelli

Dipartimento di Biopatologia Umana, Cattedra di Ematologia, Universita' «La Sapienza», Via Benevento, 6, 00161 Rome, Italy

ABSTRACT

Le infezioni rappresentano la piu' frequente causa di morte nei pazienti affetti da leucemia acuta con una incidenza che va dal 37 al 69 per cento a seconda delle casistiche considerate. Il trattamento empirico precoce con antibiotici a largo spettro in caso di infezione sospetta produce una risposta clinica favorevole nel 65-75 per cento dei pazienti anche in assenza di documentazione microbiologica. Nuovi problemi stanno comunque sorgendo, legati al cambiamento delle pratiche mediche che hanno determinato l'emergenza di nuovi patogeni; i farmaci ad ampio spettro in monoterapia ovvero l'associazione di beta-lattamici, sebbene sembrino efficaci e meno tossici, non posseggono l'auspicato effetto antibatterico sinergico; l'aumento delle infezioni da germi Gram-positivi, sembra suggerire l'aggiunta della vancomicina nel trattamento empirico, ma non trova tutti gli autori concordi, come anche l'eventuale rimozione del catetere venoso centrale in caso di batteriemia legata al catetere. I lunghi periodi di immunosoppressione iatrogena sottopongono questi pazienti al rischio di episodi infettivi multipli e di superinfezioni e generano controversie sulla durata e sulle eventuali modifiche della terapia. Alla luce di quanto sopra, si desume che i principi per il trattamento delle infezioni nei pazienti affetti da malattie ematologiche maligne sono in continua evoluzione e richiedono la dedizione e l'immaginazione del medico.

KEYWORDS

Acute leukemia, neutropenia, fever, antibiotic therapy.

Infection still plays the major role in the mortality associated with leukemias and some lymphomas. This information emanates from the major cancer treatment centres and therefore represents a population in which particularly vigorous chemotherapeutic, radiotherapeutic and supportive measures have been given. Hersh et al. (1965) summarized the experience between 1954 and 1963 at the National Cancer Institute . The period analyzed by Hersh significantly contrasts with the experience reported by Levine et al.(1974) from the same institution for the period between 1965 and 1971 . Infection accounted for 38 per cent of the primary causes of death in patients with acute leukemia in the former series between 1954 and 1963, and increased up to 69 per cent in the latter series. One of the major differences between the two series was the decline of deaths primarily associated with hemorrhage. It is in fact particularly impressive that hemorrhage as the major coprimary cause of death declined at the National Cancer Institute from 31.7 per cent in the 1954-1963 observation period (Hersh, 1965) to only 10 per cent in the series reported by Levine et al.(1974). Difficulty must be acknowledged, however, in distinguishing between the roles of infection and hemorrhage as causes of mortality, since a good number of infectious processes can trigger disseminated intravascular coagulation and, conversely, a site where bleeding has occurred can become a focus for infection. In the Levine series,(1974) infection alone appears to account for almost 70 per cent of deaths in the above patients. Since hemorrhage and infections together represent another 10 per cent, it seems reasonable to attribute some 75-80 per cent of deaths in patients with acute leukemia to infection-related causes (Young, 1988).

This high infective mortality persists despite the progresses obtained in the management of some severe complications, such as septicemias. In fact, in the seventies the outcome of sepsis in cancer patients was dismal, particularly in those with severe neutropenia. In a classic study of gram-negative bacillary bacteremia (1962), Mc Cabe and Jackson reported a 90 per cent mortality rate in patients with "rapidly fatal" underlying illness, most of whom had neutropenia and cancer. Early on it was recognized that granulocytopenia was the major factor that predisposes cancer patients to frequent and severe sepsis. Schimpff et al.(1971) proposed the empiric treatment of granulocytopenic cancer patients with broad spectrum antibiotics as soon as fever was present. This approach ran counter to a basic principle of antimicrobial therapy which required the demonstration of the infected site as well as the pathogen before initiating antibiotics (Klastersky, 1988). Nevertheless, the fact that the mortality rate for gram-negative septicemias has nowadays decreased to 20 per cent, and may also be lower in some series, has gradually led to the general acceptance of Schimpff's principle.
In our experience letality for sepsis decreased from 60 per cent in 1980 to 20 per cent in 1984 (Martino, 1985a).
New problems are however emerging, still with life threatening implications. Changing medical practices contribute to the emergence of new pathogens, and new drug developments offer new

treatment options as well as sources for controversy. We shall try to thoroughly evaluate the following questions, whenever possible within the framework of controlled clinical trials.

EMPIRIC ANTIMICROBIAL TREATMENT : WHICH PATIENTS NEED IT ?

A pragmatic approach is to set an antimicrobial treatment relying upon the best available informations and to adjust therapy as soon as the results of specific laboratory tests return. If neither objective findings of infection nor any clinical changes suggestive of microbial infection are present rather than fever secondary to the underlying malignancy, most authors (Rubin,1988) agree upon treating the febrile patient whenever the underlying disease is worsening and/or the neutrophil count is falling. Bodey et al. (1966) established that the infective risk is definitely increased in patients with less than 500 neutrophils per cubic millimeter .In a recent study (Martino, 1985b) we have observed that 239 out of 262 patients (91.2%) with a neutrophil count below 100 per cubic millimeter had at least one infective episode; furthermore 65 out of 127 patients (51.2%) with a neutrophil count between 100 and 499 per cubic millimeter had also a minimum of one infective episode .

The risk of infection is also correlated to the duration of neutropenia. In one of our studies, (Giunchi, 1985) 275 patients who did not develop infection had a mean duration of neutropenia of 2.2 days, whereas 278 patients who did develop infection had a mean duration of neutropenia of 13.2 days (neutropenia below 500 neutrophils per cubic millimeter).

Even if the number of normal neutrophils exceeds 1000 per cubic millimeter, the sudden fall in the white blood cells count induced by cytotoxic drugs will virtually ensure the patient to become functionally aplastic within a matter of days. Therefore, the sudden appearance of fever and findings suggestive of septicemia, such as hyperventilation, acidosis, hypotension and hypovolemia would be decisive factors in opting for antimicrobial treatment. On the other hand, if the patient's white blood cells count is low but is also slowly rising, and bone marrow examination reveals repopulation with normal morphological elements, we would be less inclined in being aggressive about antibacterial treatment in the setting of low-grade fever. EORTC Trial I (Klastersky, 1988) showed that the response to antimicrobial courses was 36 per cent when the initial granulocyte count of 500 per cubic millimeter was decreasing along the treatment and it was a good 87 per cent whenever the initial count was gradually increasing.

ANTIBIOTIC TREATMENT : WHEN TO START ?

In 1971 Armstrong et al. observed that 43 per cent of deaths in patients with acute leukemia were due to Gram-negative rod bacteremias: out of these, 73 per cent were sustained by

Pseudomonas aeruginosa. Furthermore, in 60 per cent of cases, the above pathogen caused death within just 48 hours. In view of the above, it is stated that the treatment must be started as soon as possible. Andriole (Andriole VT, communication, 6th Mediterranean Congress on Chemotherapy, 1988) reviewed 300 cases of Pseudomonas aeruginosa bacteremias, observing that the mortality rate was 34 per cent when the antimicrobial treatment was started within eight hours from fever appearance, and it raised up to 90 per cent whenever the treatment was started after eight hours.

EMPIRIC ANTIBIOTIC TREATMENT : HOW MANY ANTIBIOTICS ?

In order to enhance the efficacy of therapy, substantial evidence exists for the use of multiple antimicrobial agents as initial treatment. In addition, there is need to ensure that these agents be given in a sufficient dosage, in order to achieve adequate therapeutic levels. As far as the febrile neutropenic patients are concerned, an essential component of empirical therapy ought to be an aminoglycoside, paired with a beta-lactam agent (Rubin M 1988).By employing two agents, we not only achieve a broadering of the antibacterial spectrum, but we also take advantage of possible synergistic interactions between these agents. In fact, antimicrobial synergism between aminoglycosides and beta-lactams has been documented with in vitro experiments as well as with experimental infections (Young, 1982). As far as human Gram-negative infections are concerned, some authors have shown that the use of synergistic combinations is associated with significantly better results than with non synergistic ones. In particular, a statistically significant difference in the clinical outcome has been reported in non-neutropenic patients with various neoplasms (75 per cent of response with synergistic combinations versus 41 per cent with non synergystic ones) (Klastersky, 1977); in patients with mild neutropenia, less than 2000 polimorphonucleates per cubic millimeter (79 versus 33 per cent) (Anderson, 1978); and in patients with hematologic malignancies and severe neutropenia, less than 500 neutrophils per cubic millimeter (96 versus 54 per cent) (Martino, 1985c).

Sinergy seems to be even more important when the offending pathogen is Pseudomonas aeruginosa. In these regards, we observed (Martino, 1985c) 91 per cent of response by using a synergistic combination of antimicrobials versus a poor 22 per cent by using a non synergistic one ($p<0.001$).Conversely, as far as Escherichia coli septicemias are concerned, neither synergistic nor non synergistic combinations showed a statistically significant difference of clinical response (100 per cent versus 87 per cent).The in vitro synergy induces higher serum bactericidal levels, that are particularly effective for the favourable clinical outcome in case of severe neutropenia, as shown on table 1 (Martino 1985c).

Table 1. Relationship among peak levels of SBA, granulocyte count and clinical outcome in Gram-negative sepsis.

SBA	< 100 PMN/mm^3		100-500 PMN/mm^3	
	No.	% Response	No.	% Response
<1:16	20	15*^	12	66*#
>1:16	30	92^	12	100#

^* p<0.005; #= not significant
SBA= Serum Bactericidal Activity

In view of the above, it seems that synergistic combinations are mandatory when the patient is profoundly granulocytopenic (<100 polimorphonucleates per cubic millimeter), or else when the organisms' sensitivity to single antimicrobials is poor (i.e. Pseudomonas aeruginosa).

There is a persistent debate about the relative merits of agents within the aminoglycoside class and whether the beta-lactam agent should be a cephalosporin, an antipseudomonal penicillin, or else one of the newer compounds, such as monobactams and beta-lactamase inhibitors paired with a penicillin. Many new drugs belonging to the beta-lactam class have been introduced into clinical use during the past five years; many of these agents are considerably augmented in their Gram-negative coverage. Nonetheless, a consistent finding has been a relative decrease in antistaphilococcal activity. Some classes of new compounds, such as the monobactams, completely lack Gram-positive activity and cannot therefore be used alone in empirical therapy.

As far as the choice of the beta-lactam is concerned, there will be no clear cut regimen that most investigators and clinicians would consider ideal, because of the local epidemiology of the different institutions. Cefotaxime, for instance, the first of the third-generation cephalosporins, has markedly augmented activity against many important Gram-negative rods such as Escherichia coli and Klebsiella species; it has also been reported the clinical efficacy of cefotaxime used alone or in combination with other antimicrobials. In an open study, we observed (Martino, 1985d) 84 per cent response in the treatment of bacteremic episodes in neutropenic patients treated with the combination cefotaxime plus amikacin; in case of Pseudomonas aeruginosa bacteremia, the response rate was 62 per cent. Conversely, in the same period, EORTC studies (Klastersky, 1986) showed poor results with the very same combination, partially because of deficiencies in activity against Pseudomonas species. EORTC Trial IV (1987) compared ceftazidime plus a short course of amikacin (three days), with ceftazidime plus a full course of amikacin (at least nine days). In patients with Gram-negative bacillary bacteremia, the latter course was associated with a higher response rate, as compared with the former (81 per cent versus 40 per cent, p<0.002). These results seem to suggest that the combination of ceftazidime plus amikacin, given in a full course, might be more advantageous. On the other hand, Pizzo et al. (1986) reported favourable results in granulocytopenic cancer patients by using ceftazidime alone; however, their study was performed in less severely neutropenic patients with a predominance of young individuals affected by lymphomas or solid tumors rather than by acute leukemias. In addition, their protocol allowed for very early addition of other antibiotics, and these instances were not classified as failures. They concluded that ceftazidime alone was as effective as a triple drug regimen (carbenicillin plus cephalotin and gentamicin). They however indicated that in Gram-negative bacillary bacteremias these directories should be cautiously applied, and that the emergence of resistance to the beta-lactam antibiotic should be carefully monitored for. Finally, in Pizzo's study, conditions, in which the usefulness of synergism is proven, were lacking .

The advisability of including an antistaphilococcal agent in the initial empirical combination of antibiotics represents another main question. Gram-positive coccal bacteremias have become over the years more prevalent and the response rate of these infections to empirical antibiotic regimens has progressively decreased from 80 to 42 per cent (Klastersky, 1988).

As shown on fig.1, Gram-positive bacteremias increased from 10 to 62 per cent of the overall sepsis occurred over the span of fifteen years in neutropenic patients attending the Institute of Hematology of the University "La Sapienza" of Rome.

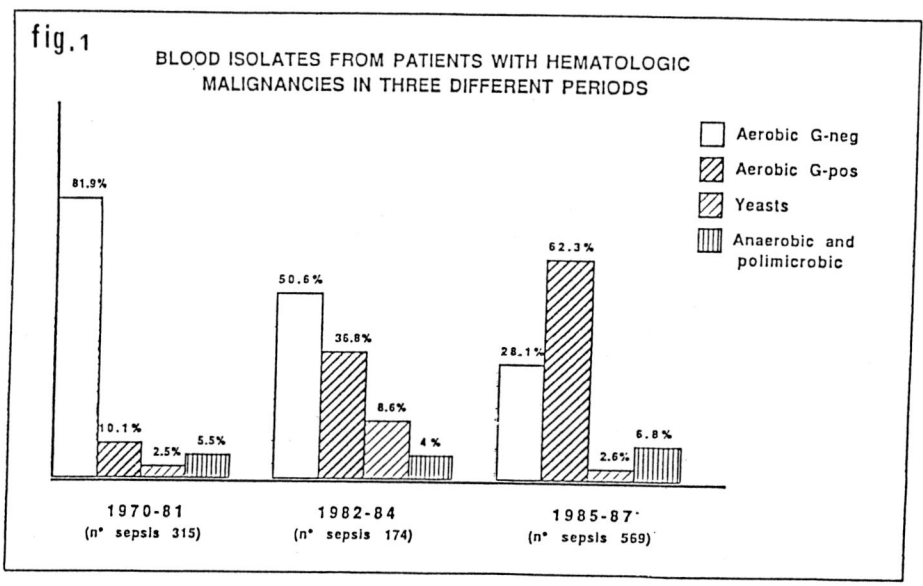

Whether specific empiric antistaphylococcal therapy is necessary, is still controversial. Some authors have observed good results by adding vancomycin or else teicoplanin to empirical therapy (Karp, 1986; Del Favero, 1987); other authors, with retrospective studies, did not find statistical differences (Mark Rubin, 1988). Citing Robert Rubin,(1988) Gram-positive infections, due to the surprisingly low mortality rate (4 per cent) may be approached as "diagnostic dilemmas rather than therapeutic emergencies".
In conclusion, many important questions still remain completely or partially unsettled, including the optimal duration of empirical therapy and its relationship with the occurrence of secondary as well as nonbacterial superinfections.
Principles for management of infections are continuing to evolve, but some methodologic approaches are actually established: the empiric therapy should be early started in the setting of profound granulocytopenia; the antimicrobial combination should include an anti-pseudomonal beta-lactam plus an aminoglycoside, potentially synergistic.

REFERENCES

Anderson, E.T. (1978): Antimicrobial synergism in the therapy of Gram-negative bacteremia. Chemotherapy 24, 45-54.
Armstrong, D (1971): Infectious complications of neoplastic diseases. Med.Clin.North Am. 55, 729-745.
Bodey,G.P. (1966): Quantitative relationships between circulating leukocytes and infection in patients with acute leukemia. Ann.Int.Med. 64, 328-340.
Del Favero, A. (1987): Prospective randomized clinical trial of teicoplanin for empiric combined antibiotic therapy in febrile, granulocytopenic acute leukemia patients. Antimicr.Ag.Chemother. 31, 1126-9.
EORTC (1987): Ceftazidime combined with a short or long course of amikacin for empirical therapy of Gram-negative bacteremia in cancer patients with granulocytopenia. N.Engl.J.Med. 317, 1612-1618.
Giunchi, G. (1985): Le infezioni nei pazienti neutropenici. In Relazione all'86 Congresso della Societa' Italiana di Medicina Interna. pp.433-523. Roma: L.Pozzi Press.
Hersh, E.M. (1965): Causes of death in acute leukemia. J.A.M.A. 193, 105-109.
Karp, JE (1986): Empiric use of vancomycin during prolonged treatment-induced granulocytopenia. Randomized double-blind, placebo-controlled clinical trial in patients with acute leukemia. Am J Med 81,237-242.
Klastersky, J. (1977): Significance of antimicrobial synergism for the outcome of Gram-negative sepsis. Am.J.Med.Sci. 273, 157-167.
Klastersky, J. (1986): Prospective randomized comparison of three antibiotic regimens for empirical therapy of suspected bacteremic infections in febrile granulocytopenic patients. Antimicrob.Ag.Chemother. 29, 263-270.

Klastersky, J. (1988): Empiric antimicrobial therapy for febrile granulocytopenic cancer patients: lessons from four EORTC trials. Eur.J.Cancer Clin.Oncol. 24s, 35-45.
Levine, A.S. (1974): Hematologic malignancies and other marrow failure states: progress in the management of complicating infections. Semin.Hematol. 11, 141-202.
Martino, P. (1985a): Water supply as a source of Pseudomonas aeruginosa in a Hospital for Hematological malignancies. Boll.Ist.Sieroter.Milan. 64, 2.
Martino, P. (1985b): Superinfections during antimicrobial treatment with Betalactam-aminoglycoside combinations in neutropenic patients with hematologic malignancies. Infection 13s, 115-122.
Martino, P. (1985c): Serum bactericidal activity as a therapeutic guide in severely granulocytopenic patients with Gram-negative sepsis. Eur. J. Cancer Clin. Oncol. 21, 439-445.
Martino, P. (1985d): Cefotaxime plus amikacin as empir therapy in the treatment of febrile episodes in neutropenic patients with hematologic malignancies. Infection 13, 125-129.
Mc Cabe, W.R. (1962): Gram-negative bacteremia II. Clinical, laboratory and therapeutic observations. Arch.Intern.Med. 110, 856-864.
Pizzo, P.A. (1986): A randomized trial comparing ceftazidime alone with combination antibiotic therapy in cancer patients with fever and neutropenia. N.EnglJ.Med. 315, 552-558
Rubin, M. (1988): Gram-positive infections and use of vancomycin in 550 episodes of fever and neutropenia. Ann.Int.Med. 108, 30-35.
Rubin, R. (1988): Empiric antibacterial therapy in granulocytopenia induced by cancer chemotherapy. Ann.Int.Med. 108, 134-136.
Schimpff, (1971): Empiric therapy with carbenicillin and gentamicin for febrile patients with cancer and granulocytopenia. N.Engl.J.Med. 284, 1061-1064.
Young, L.S. (1982): Combination or single drug therapy for Gram-negative sepsis. In Current clinical topics in infectious diseases, Vol.3, ed J.S.Remington M.N.Swartz, pp 177-205. New York: McGraw-Hill Press.
Young, L.S. (1988): Management of infections in leukemia and lymphoma. In Clinical approach to infection in the compromised host, 2nd edn, ed R.H.Rubin and L.S.Young, pp 467-501. New York and London: Plenum Medical Book Company.

RESUME

Les infections representent encore aujourd'houi la complication mortelle la plus frequente chez les malades affectes par leucemie aigue. Le traitement empirique precoce de la fièvre avec des antibiotiques ayant un large spectre d'activitée, produit un succes clinique dans 65-75 per cent des cas, même sans une precise documentation microbiologique. On observe malgré tout,

l'apparition de nouveaux problèmes et la poussée de nouvelles étiologies liées aux changements des pratiques thérapeutiques. L'utilisation d'un antibiotique puissant en monothérapie semble aussi efficace et moins toxique des combinaisons d'une betalactamine avec un aminioglicoside, mais toutefois depourvue d'effet synergique; les plus fréquentes infections à bacterie Gram-positive semblent conseiller l'utilization empirique de la vancomicine mais les auteurs ne sont pas tous d'accord.
L'immunodepression prolongée provoquée par les medicament antitumeur peux conduir au risque des infections et des superinfections: les auteurs ne sont pas tous d'accord sur la durée de la thérapie. En conclusion les principes qui determinent le traitement des infections chez les malades atteints de leucemie aigüe continuent a changer; ils ont besoin du dévouement et de l'imagination du medicin.

Infections and haemorrhage in acute leukaemia, T. Barbui, A. Falanga, B. Minetti, S. Gorini, G. Tognoni and M.D. Donati, eds. John Libbey Eurotext, Paris © 1989, pp. 195-199

A randomized study comparing imipenem-cilastatin to ceftazidime and amikacin for the treatment of infections in acute leukemia patients. Preliminary results

G. Capnist, T. Chisesi, A. Vaglia[1], I. Piacentini[2], G. Pellizzari, E. Dini

Department of Hematology, [1] of Infectious Diseases and [2] Microbiology, S. Bortolo Hospital, Vicenza, Italy

ABSTRACT

Between October, 1987 and April 1988 40 leukopenic patients with acute leukemia during remission induction treatment were assigned at random to receive either Imipenem (I):1g every 6 hours, or Ceftazidime:2g every 8 hours plus Amikacin (CA): 500mg every 8 hours for 40 fever episodes. A total of 17 courses of I and 23 of CA therapy were given.
The evaluation of response was made at 72 hours without modification of the regimen.
The overall response rate of infections treated with I alone was 65% and 56% in those who received the combination. In the bacteriologically proven infections the response rate was 67% and 75% respectively. Four out of 5 gram negative bacillemias treated with I and 4 out of 8 by the combination were cured. Seven out of 10 gram positive bacillary septicaemias responde to I alone, 2/5 to the combination. Nine pneumonitis were recorded and have been cured by I alone in 2/4 cases and in 1/5 patients by the combination. Seven fungal infections were suspected but not proven: 5 of them improved or were cured by an early empiric Amphotericin B therapy. The rate of superinfections and toxicity were very low. Two infection related deaths were recorded. No resistant organisms to I were isolated; on the contrary Ceftazidime resistant isolates were 5/16(35%) and Amikacin resistant bacteria 3/15(20%). In conclusion these initial findings led to us to consider Imipenem at least as effective as the combination of Ceftazidime and Amikacin and to carry on the study.

KEY WORDS: Acute leukemia, antibiotic therapy.

INTRODUCTION

Considerable interest has been generated by the new extended spectrum antibiotic Imipenem-Cilastatin (Barza,1983; Geddes, 1985; Leuthy, 1983; Remington, 1984; Calandra, 1988). Clinical trials have established its efficacy and safety, but there are few experiences with this antibiotic in cancer patients (Calandra, 1984)

either as primary (Bodey, 1986; Bodey, 1987; Baruchel, 1986) or secondary therapy (Bodey, 1986).
In vitro studies conducted by our unit had shown its broad spectrum activity, giving the possibility of devising antibiotic regimen without an aminoglycoside. The antibiotic regimen previously used at our department for febrile acute leukemia patients was Ceftazidime plus Netilmicin: that combination had proved satisfactory (Capnist, 1987). We present here a schedule comparing Imipenem alone with Ceftazidime plus Amikacin in neutropenic leukemia patients during induction treatment.

MATERIALS AND METHODS

Between October, 1987 and April, 1988 40 neutropenic (< 100 per mm3) patients with acute leukemia during remission induction treatment entered the study.
The patients details are given in Table 1.

Table 1. Characteristics of study patients

Characteristics	I	CA
Number of patients	17	23
Age (yr)	43	39
Sex (f/m)	9/8	15/9
Diagnosis		
AML 1 induction	5	10
AML 2 induction	10	6
ALL 1 induction	2	5
ALL 2 induction	0	2
<100 PMNS/mm3(days)	13	14
Central venous catheter	10	14

Neutropenic patients were elegible if they developed a temperature $>38C$. not associated with the administration of pyrogenic substances (blood transfusions, immunotherapeutic agents etc.). Antibiotic prophylaxis consisted of Norfloxacin plus Ketoconazole for I and Trimethoprim-Sulfamethoxazole plus Ketoconazole for CA group. Patients were excluded from the study for any of the following reasons: history of anaphylactic reaction to other beta-lactam compounds, severe liver or renal impairments (bilirubin $>3.0mg/dl$, creatinine $> 3.0mg/dl$), or underlying central nervous system disease. Microbiologic surveillance and x-ray examination were done as previously described (Capnist, 1987).
The minimal inhibitory concentration (MIC) of I against the infecting organisms was determined with serial two-fold dilutions of the antibiotic in Muller-Hinton broth; The MIC of Ceftazidime and Amikacin was obtained as previous described (Capnist, 1987). Febrile episodes were classified as bacteriologically or clinically confirmed or fever of unknown origin(FUO).
At the onset of fever patients received Imipenem-Cilastatin: 1g every 6 hours or Ceftazidime: 2g every 8 hours plus Amikacin: 500mg every 8 hours for 40 fever episodes.
Response was defined as disappearance of all clinical and laboratory

evidence of infection after 72 hours of therapy. All responding patients were treated until the bone marrow recovered. Treatment was discontinued and other antibiotics were instituted after 72 hours in non responding patients or if the isolated organism was resistent to the antibiotics or according to clinical indication. No granulocyte transfusion were given. In case of no response to the second antibiotic regimen patients persistently febrile underwent Amphotericin B 1mg/day.

RESULTS

A total of 17 courses of I and 23 of CA therapy were given. Patients in I group needed parenteral antibiotics during 65% of the days they were granulocytopenic compared to 96% of these days in CA group. The overall results are presented in Table 2:

Table 2. Response according to therapeutic regimen

	I		CA		TOT
	episodes	resp(%)	episodes	resp(%)	resp(%)
Total	17	11(65)	23	13(56)	24(60)
FUO	2	2	7	5	7
Clinical i.	6	1	8	3	4
Microbiological i.	12	8	12	9	17(71)

the response rate was 60%, 65% and 56% for I and CA group respectively. The response rate was higher in the 17 episodes in which the pathogen was known (71% vs 48%). The majority of fevers of unknown origin occurred in patients who received CA therapy after TS prophylaxis. Clinical and microbiological infections occurred with the same frequency in both groups. The low response rate among the clinical infections depended on the high number of pneumonias (Table 3) furthermore seven of them received empirically Amphotericin B because of suspected fungal infection.

Table 3. Results by site of infection

	I		CA	
	episodes	resp(%)	episodes	resp(%)
Bacteremia	12	8(67)	12	9(75)
Pneumonitis	4(3)*	2	5(3)*	1
Soft tissue	2	0	4(2)*	4
Urinary tract	1(1)*	1	0	0

*in parentheses number of infections with associated bacteremia

The organisms causing septicaemias were 15 in I and 13 in CA treated patients: in the former group most of them resulted G+; on the contrary G- resulted the most frequent in the latter group. The responses according to infecting organism in septicaemia are shown in Table 4. I resulted clearly superior than the combination (73% vs 46%) either against G+ or G-. No resistant organisms to I were isolated. Ceftazidime resistant

organisms resulted 5/15 and Amikacin resistant bacteria 3/15.
No patients developed allergic reaction to I its most common side effect was nausea. Renal and hepatic toxicity were not observed. There were 2 infections related deaths, 1 per group.

Table 4. Response rate in septicaemias

	I		CA	
	episodes	resp	episodes	resp
Gram -negative				
Klebsiella	1	1	0	0
Escherichia coli	1	1	5	3
Pseudomonas a.	3	2	2	0
flavobacterium	0		1	1
Gram-positive				
Staphylococci	5	3	3	1
Streptococci	4	3	2	1
Corynebacterium	1	1	0	0

DISCUSSION

Imipenem has been found to be a useful antibiotic for single agent therapy of most infections in cancer patients (Bodey, 1986; Bodey, 1987; Baruchel, 1986) either as initial (Bodey, 1987) or when used as secondary therapy among patients with documented infections who failed to respond to other antibiotics (Bodey, 1986).

An in vitro evaluation of this drug at our department had shown an excellent activity against gram-negative and positive organisms. Since the former pathogens were the most common in our previous experience but an emergence of the latter was evident (Capnist, 1987), a clinical evaluation of this compound was undertaken, comparing it to Ceftazidime and Amikacin. In this study the cure rate for patients receiving I alone was equal to or quite superior than the rates obtained in those receiving the combination.

All the patients had received two different antibiotic prophylaxis and that provoked a different incidence in G+ and G- organisms in the two groups. Nevertheless I alone resulted more effective than the combination either against G+ or G- bacteria: the poorest response rate in this study was among infections caused by Pseudomonas aeruginosa and pneumonitis both in Ceftazidime and Amikacin group. I proved to be highly effective for a broad range of organisms.

No resistant organisms to I were isolated; on the contrary Ceftazidime resistant isolates resulted 5/15 and to Amikacin 3/15.

In conclusion Imipenem seems to be at least as effective as the combination of Ceftazidime and Amikacin. Continued study is ongoing at this center to confirm these early results obtained between October, 1987 and April, 1988.

Baruchel,A.,Hartmann,O., Andremont,A., Tancrede,C.(1986):Severe Gram negative infections in neutropenic children cured by imipenem/cilastatin in combination with aminoglycoside. J.Antimicrob. Chemother. 18, suppl.E, 161-166.

Barza,M.(1984):Imipenem:A new carbapenem antibiotic. Eur.J.Clin.Microbiol. 3, 453-497.

Bodey,G.P., Alvarez,M.E.,Paula,G.J., Rolston,K.V.I., Steelhammer,L.,Fainstein,V.(1986):Imipenem-Cilastatin as initial therapy for febrile cancer patients.Antimicrob. Agents and Chemother. 30, 2, 211-214.

Bodey,G.P., Elting,L., Jones,P., Alvarez,M.E., Rolston,K., Fainstein,V.(1987): Imipenem-Cilastatin therapy of infections in cancer patients. Cancer 60, 255-262.

Bodey,G.P., Rolston,K., Jones,P., Alvarez,M.E., Fainstein,V., Steelhammer,L. (1986):Imipenem/Cilastatin as secondary therapy for infections in cancer patients. J.Antimicrob. Chemother. 18, Suppl.E, 161-166.

Calandra,G.B., Ricci,F.M., Wang,C., Brown,K.R.(1988):The efficacy results and safety profile of Imipenem/Cilastatin from the clinical Research trials. J.Clin.Pharmacol. 28, 120-127.

Calandra,G.B., Hesney,M., Grad,C.(1984):A multiclinic randomized study ot the comparative efficacy, safety and tolerance of Imipenem/Cilastatin and Moxalactam. Eur. J. Clin. Microbiol. 3, 478-487.

Capnist,G., Chisesi T., Vaglia,A., Piacentini,I., Battista,R., D'Emilio,A., Vespignani,M., Dini,E.(1987): Sequential antibiotic therapy in acute leukemia. Haematologica 72, 439-444.

Geddes,A.M., Stille,W.(1985):Imipenem:The first thienamycin antibiotic. Rev. Infect. Dis. 3, S353-S356.

Leuthy,R., New,H.C., Phillips,I.(1983):A perspective on Imipenem. J.Antimicrob.Chemother. 12, Suppl.D, 1-156.

Remington, J.S.,(1985): Carbapenems: A new class of Antibiotics. 78, Suppl.6A, 1-167.

Preliminary evaluation of ofloxacin (OFL), a new fluorinated quinolone, versus trimethoprim/sulfamethoxazole (TMP/SMZ) in prophylaxis of infections in leukemic patients

R. Fanci, A. Bosi, G. Longo, A. Bartolini[1], D. Aquilini[1], A. Orsi[2], P. Rossi Ferrini, F. Paradisi[1]

Cattedra e Divisione di Ematologia, [1] Cattedra di Malattie Infettive, [2] Laboratorio di Batteriologia e Virologia, Universita' degli Studi ed Ospedale di Careggi, I-50134, Firenze, Italy

SUMMARY

The efficacy of OFL in preventing the bacterial infections was compared with that of TMP/SMZ in a randomized double blind trial in patients with acute leukemia undergoing induction chemotherapy. 20 pts were randomly allocated to receive orally twice a day OFL (300 mg) or TMP/SMZ (160/800 mg) in a non cross over study. The two groups were comparable for number of granulocytopenic episodes, number of days at risk of infections in aplastic phase, and for number of days of prophylactic treatment. Statistical analysis failed to show any significant difference between the 2 groups as regards number of febrile episodes, days of fever, number of documented infections and number of febrile episodes of undefined origin.

KEYWORDS

Trimethoprim/sulfamethoxazole, ofloxacin, bacterial infections, leukemia.

INTRODUCTION

Patients with acute leukemia receiving antineoplastic regimens are at enhanced risk of serious infections (Bodey, 1966). Previous studies showed that TMP/SMZ reduce the incidence of infections in granulocytopenic patients (Dekker, 1981; Rozenberg-Arska, 1983) but some disadvantages were observed: increased time of profound granulocytopenia (Pizzo, 1981), emergence of resistant microorganisms (Dekker, 1981), and increasing number of allergic reactions. The new generation of fluorinated quinolones with their broad antimicrobial activity against aerobic gram positive and gram negative bacteria (Smith, 1986), and their low activity against anaerobic bacteria have the potential for being a good alternative for prophylaxis in granulocytopenic patients. The efficacy of OFL, a new orally absorbed fluorinated quinolone, in preventing bacterial infections was compared with that of TMP/SMZ in a randomized double blind study in patients with acute leukemia undergoing induction chemotherapy.

SUBJECTS AND METHODS

From January to June 1987, 20 patients observed at Division of Hematology of the University of Florence, Italy, were randomly allocated to receive orally twice a day OFL (300 mg) or TMP/SMZ (160/800 mg) in a cross over study starting 2-3 days before the antineoplastic regimen until the recovery from the aplastic phase. All pts were afebrile, had no signs of infections, and were not receiving antibacterial agents. Statistical analysis was performed with the Mann-Whitney test.

RESULTS

The two groups were comparable for number of granulocytopenic episodes, number of days at risk of infections in aplastic phase (Table 1) and for number of days of prophylactic treatment (OFL 241 days, mean 26.1; TMP/SMZ 335, mean 33.5; p=ns).

Table 1. Granulocytopenic episodes in OFL and TMP/SMZ groups

granulocytes ($10^9/l$)		N Episodes	Days at risk	P
<0.2	OFL	14	262	ns
	TMP/SMZ	15	349	
0.2-0.5	OFL	3	66	ns
	TMP/SMZ	4	67	
>0.5	OFL	3	45	ns
	TMP/SMZ	1	10	

In TMP/SMZ patients, 11 febrile episodes were observed with a total of 43 days of fever. In OFL patients 14 febrile episodes were observed with 68 febrile days. Statistical analysis failed to show any significant difference between the 2 groups as regards number of febrile episodes, days of fever, number of documentated infections and number of febrile episodes of undefined origin (Table 2). The patogens identified in microbiologically documented infections are detailed in Table 3.

DISCUSSION

This study assessed the efficacy of ofloxacin respect to TMP/SMZ in preventing the bacterial infections in neutropenic patients with acute leukemias. The classic studies of Dekker (1981) and Rozenberg-Arska (1983)

Table 2. Analysis of febrile episodes in OFL and TMP/SMZ patients

	OFL	TMP/SMZ	P
N of neutropenic episodes	20	20	ns
N of febrile episodes	14	11	ns
% febrile episodes/neutropenic ep	70	55	ns
N days with fever	68	43	ns
N days at risk	373	426	ns
% days with fever/days at risk	18.2	10	ns
Documentated infections			
with bacteraemia	3	7	ns
without bacteraemia	1	1	ns
Possible clinical infections	5	0	ns
Fever of undefined origin	5	4	ns

Table 3. Microbiologically documented infections: all pathogens

	Number of isolates	Bacteraemia
OFLOXACIN (*)	5	3
Ps. stutzeri	1	1
Staph. aureus	1	1
Staph. coagulase neg.	1	0
Str. A	1	0
Propionibacterium acnes	1	1
TMP/SMZ	8	7
Esch. coli	3	3
Ps. acidovorans	1	1
Ps. vesicularis	1	1
Staph. coagulase neg.	1	1
Staph. aureus	1	0
Str. A	1	1

(*) 1 case with multiple pathogens

showed that TMP/SMZ reduce the incidence of infections in granulocytopenic patients. In our experience the new fluorinated quinolone Ofloxacin appeared as an effective agent in preventing infections in leukemic patients in aplastic phase of antineoplastic regimens. In fact OFL resulted effective as the classic TMP/SMZ. However must be stressed that quinolones are not indicated in pediatric patients because affect bone and cartilago syntesis and they are ineffective against Pneumocystis carinii. Moreover emergence of resistant microorganisms is possible. In conclusion the results reported here show that Ofloxacin can be employed safely as alternative to TMP/SMZ for preventing infections in leukemic patients undergoing antineoplastic regimens.

REFERENCES

Bodey, G. P. (1966): Quantitative relationships between circulating leukocytes and infections in patients with acute leukemia. Ann. Int. Med. 64, 328-35.

Dekker, A.W. (1981): Prevention of infections by trimethoprim-sulfamethoxazole plus amphotercin B in patients with acute non lymphocytic leukemia. Ann. Int. Med. 95, 555-63.

Pizzo, P. A. (1981): Infections complications in the child with cancer. Management of specific infections organisms. J. Pediatr. 9, 513-20.

Rozenberg-Arska, M. (1983): Colistin and trimethoprim-sulfamethoxazole for the prevention of infection in patients with acute non lymphocytic leukemia. Decrease in the emergence of resistant bacteria. Infection 11, 167-77.

Smith, G. M. (1986): Preliminary evaluation of ciprofloxacin, a new 4-quinolone antibiotic, in the treatment of febrile neutropenic patients. J. Antimicrob. Chemother. 18 (Suppl D), 165-74.

Infection prophylaxis in acute leukemia: a comparison of norfloxacin with trimethoprim-sulfamethoxazole. Preliminary results

G. Capnist, T. Chisesi, I. Piacentini[1], A. Vaglia[2], G. Pellizzari, E. Dini

Department of Hematology of [1] Microbiology, and [2] Infectious Diseases, S. Bortolo Hospital, Vicenza, Italy

ABSTRACT

A prospective randomized study was undertaken in neutropenic patient to evaluate the effect of prophylactic Norfloxacin(N) versus Trimethoprim-Sulfamethoxazole(TS) on infection and fever rate. Fifty-two patients with acute leukemia randomly received either N:400mg bid (26 patients) or TS:160/800mg bid (26 patients) for the period of expected neutropenia. The mean duration of aplasia was 13 days for TS and 10.6 days for N group of patients. The total number of acquired infections was 20 in the N and 20 in the TS group: 12 bacteremias, 4 pneumonias and 1 infection related deaths were recorded either in the quinolone group or in TS group. Suspected fungal infection occurred in 3 N patients and in 7 who received TS prophylaxis. Patients in the N group needed parenteral antibiotics during 65% of the days they were granulocytopenic compared to 96% of these days in TS group. The isolated organisms showed a higher resistance rate to TS(81%) than to N(36%). From this preliminary results the two regimens showed no difference in the number and type of acquired infections; on the contrary the TS group had 1) and increased duration of the granulocytopenic period 2) needed more days of antibiotic therapy. 3) had a higher rate of pulmonary infiltrates and 4) a remarkable number of TS resistant organisms was isolated.

KEY WORDS: Acute leukemia, antibiotic prophylaxis.

INTRODUCTION

The greatest experience has been amassed with Trimethoprim-Sulfamethoxazole (Enno, 1978; Armstrong, 1984; Pizzo, 1983; Sharon, 1984; Gurwith, 1979; Kaufman, 1983; Gualtieri, 1983; Kramer, 1984; Wade, 1981; Zinner, 1983). The usefulness ascribed to this prophylactic therapy has variable (Sharon, 1984), some studies showing a decrease in infectious episodes (Enno, 1978; Armstrong, 1984; Pizzo, 1983; Sharon, 1984; Gurwith, 1979; Kaufman, 1983; Gualtieri, 1983) while others did not (Kramer, 1984; Wade, 1981; Zinner, 1983). In our previous experience we were not able to draw reliable information because of the lack of a control group (Capnist, 1987). Since Norfloxacin administration is associated with suppression of the gastrointestinal tract colonization by aerobic bacteria without elimination of the anaerobic flora (Karp, 1986), a prospective study was undertaken to compare the effect of prophylactic Norfloxacin (N) versus Trimethoprim-Sulfamethoxazole (TS) on infection and fever rate.

MATERIALS AND METHODS

Between October, 1987 and April, 1988 all patients over the age of 16, hospitalized at the Department of Hematology, S.Bortolo Hospital, Vicenza, Italy, who had had the diagnosis of acute leukemia either myelocitic or lymphocytic were elegible for this study. Patients underwent induction chemotherapy and were expected to develop severe neutropenia. Special isolation precautions were not employed.
Prophylactic Regimen. Patients randomly received either Norfloxacin: 400mg bid or Trimethoprim-Sulfamethoxazole: 160/800mg bid, throughout the entire period of chemotherapy.
All hospitalized patients received Ketoconazole 400mg/day. The following parameters were considered: absolute neutrophil count, temperature greather than 38 C. and occurrence of documented infections. Surveillance cultures, x-ray examination and microbiologic studies were performed as previously described (Capnist, 1987). Patients with fever after the coltures were obtained, received broad spectrum antibiotics (Ceftazidime + Amikacin the TS group or Imipenem the N treated patients).

RESULTS

Fifty-two patients were enrolled until now into the study: 26 were randomized to receive N and 26 TS. The characteristics of the patients are summerized in Table 1.

Table 1. Characteristics of study patients

Characteristics	TS	N
Number of patients	26	26
Age (yr)	42	44
Sex (f/m)	16/10	12/14
Diagnosis		
AML 1 induction	13	10
AML 2 induction	6	10
ALL 1 induction	5	5
ALL 2 induction	2	1
<100 PMNS/mm3 (days)	13.3	10.6
Central venous catheter	53%	46%

The two groups resulted homogeneous as regards age, sex, underlying disease, use of central venous catheter. The mean number of days of neutropenia was 13.3 for TS and 10.6 for N group.
Patients who received TS needed parenteral antibiotics during 96% of the days they were granulocytopenic compared to 65% of the N group.

No differences were recorded in number and site of infections (Table 2).

Table 2. Site of infections

Infection	TS	N
Bacteremia	12	12
Pneumonitis *	4(3)	4(3)
Urinary tract	0	1(1)
Soft tissue	4(1)	3
Total	20(4)	20(4)

Note: numbers in parentheses indicate number of infection with associated bacteremia. *Clinical Infection.

The incidence of gram positive infections (Table 3) resulted higher in N than in TS group (11 vs 5).

Table 3. Organisms that caused infections

Organism	TS	N
Gram-negative bacilli		
Klebsiella	0	1
Escherichia coli	5	1
Proteus spp	0	0
Pseudomonas spp	2	3
Flavobacterium	1	0
Total	8	5
Gram-positive cocci		
Streptococci	2	3
Staphylococci	3	6
Corynebacterium	0	1
Peptostreptococcus	0	1
Total	5	11

Gram negative were 8 in TS and 5 in N treated patients. No pulmonary aspergillosis were recorded, but 7 patients in TS and 3 in N group received Amphotericin B empirically for suspected fungal infections. No toxicity were noted either in TS or in N arm. Two infections related deaths occurred during the course of the study, one in the group that received TS, one in the other group.

DISCUSSION

Many studies have demonstrated TS superiority in preventing infections in cancer patients as compared to placebo (Gualtieri, 1983), no treatment (Gurwith, 1979; Kaufman, 1983) or Malidixic acid (Wade, 1981). FRACON plus TS appeared superior them FRACON alone (Enno, 1978). However its effectiveness is still an open question (Sharon, 1984). Our previous policy considered TS prophylaxis in acute leukemia patients who underwent induction remission therapy: because of the lack of a control group we were not able to drow reliable conclusion about its efficacy (Capnist, 1987).Because that in October, 1987 a randomized prospective study comparing TS prophylaxis to Norfloxacin has been started. The preliminary results shows no difference in the number and site of infection and related deaths. The isolated organisms are quite different in the two arms, G+ resulting more frequent in N group while G- did in TS group. The patients treated with TS prophylaxis experienced an increased duration of the granulocytopenic period, an increased need for intravenous antibiotics and more patients in TS group received Amphotericin B empirically than in N group. Most of the microbiological infections were caused by bacteria resistant to TS. Continuing the study is required for statistically significant results and finally conclusions.

REFERENCES

Armstrong, D.(1984):Protected environments are disconforting and expensive and not offert meaningfull protection.Am.J. Med. 76, 685-687.

Capnist,G., Chisesi, T.,Vaglia,A., Piacentini,I.,Battista,R.,Vespignani,M.,D'Emilio,A., Dini,E.(1987):Trimethoprim/Sulfamethoxazole plus Ketoconazole prophylaxis in acute leukemia.Haematologica 72, 157-161.

Enno,A.,Darrel,J., Hows,J., Catovsky,D., Goldman,J.M., Galton,D.A.G.(1978): Co-trimoxazole for prevention of infection in acute leukaemia.Lancet ii,395-7.

Gualtieri,R.J., Donowitz,G.R., Keiser,D.L., Hess,C.E., Sande,M.A.(1983):Double blind ramdomized study of prophylactic trimethoprim/sulfamethoxazole in granulocytopenic patients with hematologic malignances.Am.J. Med. 74, 934-940.

Gurwith,M.J., Brunton,J.L., Lank,B.A., Harding,G.K.M., Ronald,A.R.(1979): A prospective controlled investigation of prophylactic trimethoprim/sulfamethoxazole, in hospitalized granulocytopenic patients.Am. J. Med. 66, 248-256.

Karp,J.E., Merz,W.G., Hendricksen,C., Laughon,B., Redden,T., Bamberger,B.J., Bartlett,J.G.,Saral,R., Burke,P.J.(1986):Infection management during antileukemia treatment induced granulocytopenia:The role for oral Norfloxacin prophylaxis against infections arising from the gastrointestinal tract.Scan.J.Infect. Dis. 48, 66-78.

Kaufman,C.A., Liepman,M.K., Bergman,A.G., Mioduszewski,J.(1983):Trimethoprim /Sulfamethoxazole prophylaxis in neutropenic patients.Am.J.Med. 74, 597-604.

Kramer, B.S.,Carr,D.J., Rand,K.H., Pizzo,P.A., Hohnson,A., Robichaud,K.J., Yucha,J.B.(1984):Prophylaxis of fever and infection in adult cancer patients. Cancer 53, 329-335.

Pizzo,P.A., Schimpff,S.C.(1983):Strategies for the prevention of infections in the myelosuppressed or immunosuppressed cancer patients.Cancer Treat.Rep. 67,223-34.

Sharon,A.E.(1984):Chemoprophylaxis of bacterial infections in granulocytopenic patients.Am.J. Med. 76? 645-650.

Wade,J.C., Schimpff,S.C., Hargadon,M.T., Fortner,C.L., Young,V.M.,Wiernik,P.H. (1981)/A comparison of Trimethoprim/Sulfamethoxazole plus Nystatin with Gentamicin plus Nystatin in the prevention of infections in acute leukemia.N. Eng. J.Med. 304, 1057-1062.

Zinner,M.(1983):Prophylaxis of bacterial infections with oral antibiotics in neutropenic patients. Schweiz.Med. Wschr. 113, 7-14.

Corinebacterium JK infection in immunocompromised patient treated with teicoplanin

M. Montillo, E. Manso[1], R. Centurioni, P. Leoni, P.E. Varaldo[2]

Institutes of Clinica Medica Generale, [1] Hygiene and [2] Microbiology, University of Ancona, Medical School, Italy

Group JK corynebacteria have only recently been documented as a possible cause of serious infections in immunocompromised patients, usually those who have had extended periods of granulocytopenia as a result of hematologic malignancy (6). Moreover, Corynebacterium JK may be encountered in association with plastic indwelling catheters in patients who were not immunosupressed and did not have an underlying malignancy (4).

In these characteristics, the JK organism closely resembles coagulase-negative staphylococci; similarities also exist in regard to the resistance of both to antimicrobial therapy. JK diphteroids are resistant to most antimicrobials used in the Hospital, and vancomycin is regarded as the drug of choice.

Teicoplanin, another glycopeptide antibiotic with a mode of action and antimicrobial spectrum similar to that of vancomycin (8), has been shown to be as active in vitro as vancomycin against JK multiresistant bacteria, and may be a less toxic alternative for the treatment of JK infections (2, 7).

CASE REPORT

A 32-year-old woman received a full course of chemotherapy for Acute non Lymphoid Leukemia (ANLL). Two days after the end of treatment the patient revealed a fever and was treated empirically with ceftazidime (2 g x 3/d) and Amikacin (500 mg x 3/d). Fever remitted after 4 days but the patient developed a temperature of up to 38.9°C three days after antibiotic suspension (Figure 1).

At this time, a group JK diphteroid, only sensitive to vancomycin, teicoplanin and tetracycline grew in both of two blood cultures obtained one by venipuncture and one through a Mediport central venous catheter. A local infection at the site of catheter insertion was observed, and an abscess was drained four days later. Culture of purulence yelded JK organisms. Peripheral blood cultures became rapidly negative. Blood cultures obtained through the central venous catheter were repeatedly positive for JK, and the membrane of the removed catheter also showed a heavy growth of the organisms.

Empiric antibiotic therapy with teicoplanin (400 mg iv/d) and Amikacin (500 mg x 2/d) was initiated and fever was cleared in two days.

Three months later, in complete remission, the patient was reinfused her bone marrow cryopreserved and "ASTA-Z purged" after a superintensive chemotherapy with cyclophosphamide (50 mg/kg daily x 4 d) plus Busulfan (4mg/kg daily x 4 d).

The microbiological monitoring documented that JK group corynebacteria, isolated from rectal swab since the day preceding the operation, were subsequently isolated from various skin sites. As suggested by the multiple resistance and the identical susceptibility patterns and biochemical reactions of isolates, the same organism appeared to be involved in both rectum and skin colonization and the previous device-related bacteremia.

Owing to the appearance of fever 8 days after the transplantation (with consistently negative blood cultures), empiric therapy with teicoplanin (400 mg iv /d for two days and then 200 mg iv/d), ceftazidime (2 g x 3/d) and Amikacin (500 mg x 2/d) was started. Teicoplanin was continued for 24 days and led to complete eradication of JK colonization.

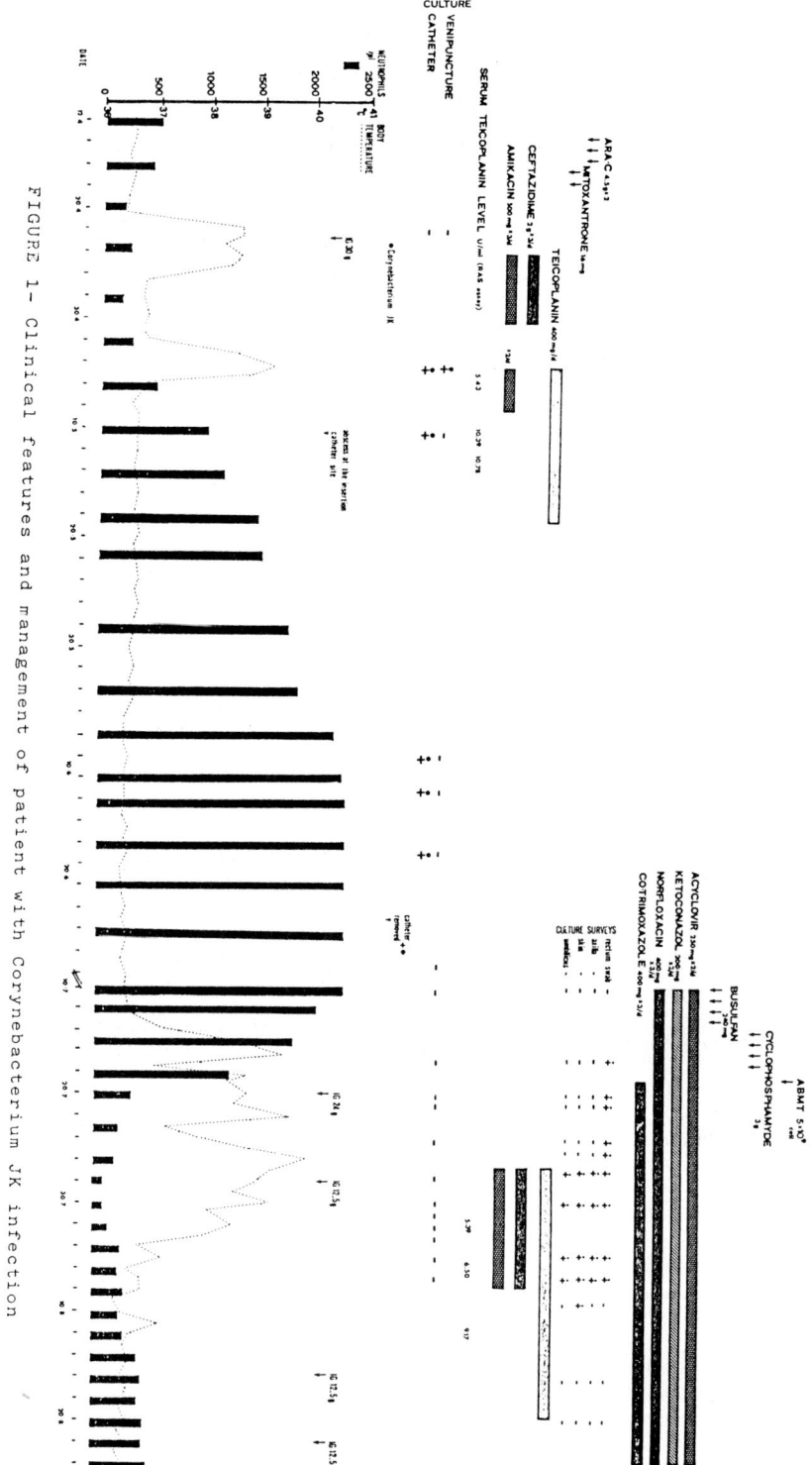

FIGURE 1- Clinical features and management of patient with Corynebacterium JK infection

MICROBIOLOGY

Corynebacterium JK was recognized by its morphologic, colonial and biochemical characteristics (1, 5). The organisms were aerobes and formed discrete, tiny, slow growing, catalase-positive colonies, non hemolitic on blood agar medium. On Gram stain it appeared as a, tiny, gram positive coccobacillus or coccus. Since JK organisms have a multiresistant susceptibility pattern as well as Group D-2 Corynebacterium, biochemical identification of isolates is needed. JK Corynebacterium are unable to produce urease, but produce acid from glucose, galactose and sometimes, as our strains, from maltose.

Antimicrobial susceptibility of all isolates tested (determined by the agar diffusion method on Mueller-Hinton Agar) showed resistance to penicillin, ampicillin, cephalotin, cefotaxime, ceftazidime, clindamycin, erythromycin, chloramphenicol, gentamycin, netilmycin and amikacin. All isolates were sensitive to vancomycin, tetracycline and teicoplanin. The MIC and MBC values of teicoplanin (determined by the broth dilution method) were of < 0.06 mg/l.

CONCLUSION

In other studies, group JK corinebacteria have been reported as the most frequent cause of bacteremia among recipients of bone marrow transplants (6); the frequency of disease due to JK organisms in this group of transplant recipients was markedly reduced when vancomycin was added to the initial empiric antibiotic regimen.

The likely source of the organism is mucocutaneous defect, such as an intravascular catheter or cellulitis.

Colonization of skin or mucosal defect frequently precedes infection; transfer from person to person seems to be the major mode of hospital spread.

As reported by others, the systemic use of vancomycin neither prevent nor control the growth of antibiotic resistant JK bacteria on the skin (3).

In our patient, however, JK skin colonization was not found after her course of teicoplanin administration.

REFERENCES

1- COYLE MB, HOLLIS DG, GROMAN NB: Corynebacterium spp. and other coryneform organisms. In EH Lennette, A Balows, WJ Hansler Jr, J Shadomy Eds. "MANUAL OF CLINICAL MICROBIOLOGY" 4th ed. American Society for Clinical Microbiology, Washington DC, pag. 193-204, 1985

2- JADEJA L, FAINSTEIN V, LEBLANC B, BODEY GP: Comparative in vitro activities of teichomycin and other antibiotic against JK diphteroids. ANTIMICHROBIAL AGENTS AND CHEMOTHERAPY 24: 145, 1983

3- LARSON EL, MCGINLEY KJ, LEYDEN JJ, COOLEY ME, TALBOT G: Skin colonization with antibiotic-resistant (JK Group)and antibiotic-sensitive lipophilic diphteroids in hospitalized and normal adults. J INFECTS DIS, 153; 701, 1986

4- RIEBEL W,FRANTZ N, ADELSTEIN D, SPAGNUOLO PJ: Corynebacterium JK: A cause of nosocomial device infection. REV INFECT DIS, 8:42, 1986

5- RILEY PS, HOLLIS DG, UTTER GB, WEAVER RE, BAKER CN: Characterization and identificatioin of 95 diphteroid (Group JK) cultures isolated from clinical specimens. J CLIN MICROBIOL, 9: 418, 1979

6- STAMM W A, TOMPKINS LS, WAGNER KF, COUNTS GW, THOMAS ED, MEYERS JD: Infection due to Corynebacterium species in marrow transplants patients. ANN INTERN MED , 91:167, 1979

7- VARALDO PE , DEBBIA E , SCHITO G: In vitro activity of teychomycin and vancomycin alone and in combination with rifampin. ANTIMICROBIALS AGENTS AND CHEMOTHERAPY , 23:402, 1983

8- WILLIAMS AH,GRUNENBER RN: Teicoplanin. J ANTIMICROB CHEMOTHER, 14:441, 1984

Relationships between serum iron levels and risk of infectious complications in acute leukemia

P.L. Garavelli

Department of Infectious Diseases. Alessandria General Hospital, Alessandria, Italy

SUMMARY

Per quanto la granulocitopenia sia il fattore di rischio più importante per l'insorgenza di complicanze infettive nei pazienti affetti da leucemia acuta, recenti indagini hanno indicato come anche la sideremia possa avere un significato prognostico aggiuntivo. Questo lavoro retrospettivo su 36 pazienti affetti da leucemia acuta non linfatica (LANL) o linfatica (LAL) conferma come valori elevati di sideremia all'esordio possano comportare un rischio maggiore di complicanze infettive da schizomiceti e/o miceti di sortita. Viene discusso il ruolo del ferro nella proliferazione dei microorganismi patogeni.

KEY WORDS: Leucemie acute, sideremia, complicanze infettive.

Opportunistic infections are an important cause of morbidity and morbility in patients with acute leukemia.
Neutropenia, due either to the replacement of normal marrow stem cells with leukemic blasts and to the cytotoxic effects of chemotherapy, is commonly recognized as the single most important prognostic factor for appearance of infectious complications.
Recent studies, however, have revealed that high serum iron levels can have an unfavourable prognostic significance in patients with acute leukemia, due to promoting effect of this ion on bacterial and yeast growth (Gordeuk,1986;Karp,1986).
To confirm these data, the possible relationships between serum iron levels at clinical presentation and subsequent development of infectious complications have been investigated.

MATERIAL AND METHODS

36 adult patients, 13 with acute lymphocytic leukemia (ALL) and 23 with acute non-lymphocytic leukemia (ANLL), admitted at the 2nd Medical Department of the University Medical Center in Pavia, have been studied.
All the patients have been treated with the same remission-inducing agents Vincristina, Cytosine Arabinoside and Daunomycin.

All the patients have been given an antibiotic coverage with trimetophrim sulfa=
metoxazole and oral nystatin from the beginning of the therapy.
In retrospective analysis, at least two episodes of hyperpyrexia in 48 hours ha=
ve been considered significative of infection; patients have divided into two
groups : those with infectious complications during remission-inducing therapy
(26 pts) and those without (10 pts).
Patients with infectious complications were started on cephalosporins and amino=
glycosides after having obtained cultures and were changed to a specific therapy
in case positive cultures.
Serum iron level has been measured with a standard colorimetric method (Bothwell,
1979).

RESULTS

Results show that in patients with infectious complications, serum iron was hi=
gher (147 ± 62 µg/dl) than in those without infection (88± 37 µg/dl) Student's
T for unpaired data gives a figure of 2.811, indicating a significant difference
at level $0.0005 < P < 0.005$.
No significant difference between the groups in granulocyte number both at begin=
ning and at chemotherapy-inducend nadir was found.
This study demonstrates that, with only one exception, a serum iron over 150µg/dl
at presentation, bears a high risk of infectious complications even if they appear
in patients with lower values.

COMMENTS

Data obtained in this study confirm that high serum iron levels can forecast an
high risk of infectious complications, in patients with acute leukemia, indepen
dent from the relevance of neutropenia.
From a biologic point of view, this relationship between body iron level and infec
tious risks has a clear interpretation.
Iron is an essential element for bacterial and yeast growth, being a fundamental
component of ribonucleotide reductase, key enzyme in DNA synthesis: to obtain the
metal, bacteria secrete molecules called Siderophora, and, having specific recep
tors, they recover these molecules from the environment after iron has been bound
(Bullen, 1978; Bullen, 1981; Neilands, 1985).
Has been demonstrated that iron containing sera stimulate growth of bacteria like
E.Coli, S.Aureus or Pseudomonas Aeruginosa, or yeasts like C.Albicans (Bullen,1981).
Transferrin, iron plasmatic carrier, is, by itself, a bacteriostatic agent becau=
se makes iron less available to microorganisms (Bothwell, 1979).
It's, however, clear, that the highest are iron levels and transferrin saturation
the most available is iron to bacterial and micotic siderophora and the easiest
for bacteria to proliferate (Pearson, 1976; Weinberg,1978; Weinberg, 1984).
In acute leukemia, serum iron increases through different mechanisms, but one is
the most important : erythropoiesis suppression and, therefore, depressed consump=
tion of transferrinic iron by erythroblasts (Bothwell, 1979).
Serum iron tends to be reduced in all the infectious and, more generally inflamma=
tory processes, because of the so called reticuloendothelial block or sideropexis
(Bothwell,1979).

Interleukin 1, produced by monocites and macrophages, stimulates ferritin synthesis inside reticuloendothelial cells, blocks iron release to-plasmatransferrin and, therefore, causes a reduction of serum iron levels.
The end result of all these events is just to reduce the serum iron available to pathogenic bacteria.
We cannot exclude that patients with acute leukemia produce less interleukin 1 and, therefore, they haven't this useful reduction of serum iron levels(Lee, 1983).
In conclusion, high levels of serum iron (150 µg/dl) in patients with acute leukemia bear an ominous prognostic significance, because they can indicate a high risk of infectious complications. Perspective studies will allow a better definition and quantification of that risk.

REFERENCES

Bothwell T.H., Charlton R.W., Cook J.D., Finch C.A.(1979): Iron metabolism in Man. Blackwell Scientific Publications, 302-3
Bullen J.J., Roger H.G., Griffiths E.(1978): Role of iron in bacterial infection. Curr.Top.Microbiol.Immunol. 80, 1-35
Bullen J.J. (1981): The significance of iron in infection. Rev.Infect.Dis. 3, 1127-38
Gordeuk V.R., Brittenham H., McLaren D., Spegnuolo P.J. (1986): Hyperferremia in immunosuppressed patients with acute non-lymphocytic leukemia and the risk of infection. J.Lab.Clin.Med. 108, 466-72
Karp J.E., Mertz W.G. (1986): Association of reduced total iron binding capacity and fungal infections in leukemic granulocytopenic patients. J.Clin.Oncol. 4, 216-20
Lee R. (1983): The anemia of chronic disease. Semin.Hematol. 20, 61-80
Neilands J.B., Nakamura K. (1985): Regulation of iron assimilation in microorganism. Nutr.Rev. 43, 193-7
Pearson H.A., Robinson J.E. (1976): The role of iron in host resistance. Adv.Pediatr. 23, 1-33
Weinberg E.D. (1978): Iron and infection. Microbiol.Rev. 42, 45-66
Weinberg E.D. (1984): Iron withholding : a defense against infection and neoplasia. Physiol. Rev. 64, 65-102.

SUMMARY

Although granulocytopenia is the major factor in the pathogenesis of infections in patients with acute leukemia, recent studies have singled out the prognostic significance of plasma iron too. This retrospective study on 36 patients with acute non-lymphocytic or lymphocytic leukemia confirms that a high plasma iron is a negative prognostic indicator for infectious complications. The role of iron in bacterial growth is examined.

KEY WORDS: Acute leukemias, serum iron levels, infectious complications.

Reproduction photomécanique
IMPRIMERIE LOUIS-JEAN
BP 87 — 05002 GAP
Tél. : 92.51.35.23
Dépôt légal : 735 — Octobre 1989
Imprimé en France